KEEPING FAITH IN MEDICINE

NAVIGATING SECULARIZED HEALTHCARE WITH GRACE AND TRUTH

DR. THEODORE K. FENSKE

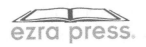

ENDORSEMENTS

"For people of faith, the integration of our faith with our vocations is a crucial and life-long task. Dr. Fenske's honest and thoughtful exploration of how his Christian faith informs the practice of medicine can aid each of us in that task. Thank you for this important and useful book."
 - **Dan Reilly,** MD, FRCPC, Obstetrics and Gynecology, Associate Clinical Professor, McMaster University

"With conscience constantly under attack, Dr. Ted Fenske's book is a much-needed analysis of how Christians should respond to the inevitable struggles that come with a secular healthcare system. Now more than ever, we need medical professionals with well-formed consciences. Now more than ever, we have need of a book like this to contextualize what is going on and where we go from here."
 - **Jonathan Van Maren,** Communications Director, Canadian Centre for Bioethical Reform

"Dr. Ted Fenske has written a book which should serve as essential reading for any Christian in the healthcare field. This is a book that addresses the controversial issues of the day with great boldness, balance and carefully considered defenses from an orthodox Christian perspective. This timely book is…from a person in the trenches who wrestles with these issues daily. If you are in the healthcare field or know someone who is, Dr. Fenske's book may be one of the most important books you could read and share with others."
 - **Dr. Arlen Salte,** Executive Director, Break Forth Ministries

"Dr. Fenske's book is must reading for university students seeking to

work as doctors, nurses and other health professionals. His deep understanding of core gospel principles, and his long-ranging experience in applying these principles in the practice of medicine, will be a source of wisdom and encouragement for students as well as for those already working in this mission field."
- **John Carpay,** B.A., LL.B., President, Justice Centre for Constitutional Freedoms

"The title seems to hint that this is just another 'How to Live your Life,' of which there are already far too many. But this book is different. Fenske invites us to walk alongside as he shares his journey through the years of medical school, residency, and early practice when he was fiercely focused on performance at every level.... Fenske articulates how this results in a loss of our identity as children of God in favor of an identity anchored in our place and position in our chosen profession. His own deeply personal story of a temporary loss of this all-consuming professional identity through sudden illness leads to his story of recovering his identity in Christ above all.... The journey concludes with a look at end-of-life issues both from the Christian view of eternal hope to the practical considerations of useful and useless treatments. This book will be a blessing to all professionals who need inspiration to refocus their lives as Christians."
- **Arnold Voth,** MD, FRCPC, Clinical Professor Internal Medicine, Royal Alexandra Hospital

"*Keeping Faith in Medicine* is the perfect prescription for medical practice today. It provides vital encouragement, solid Biblical teaching, and deeply rooted hope for Christian healers. Dr. Fenske balances patient stories, clinical experience, and accurate, practical theology as he discusses crucial issues in medicine under the overarching story of the Gospel. The title is a delightful play on words, and both senses are essential for Christian healthcare professionals as they go beyond serving well to flourishing."

- **Margaret M Cottle,** MD, CCFP (PC), Palliative Care Physician, Clinical Assistant Professor, University of British Columbia, Faculty of Medicine, Division of Palliative Care, Vancouver, BC

"Dr. Ted Fenske writes about his experience as a Christian physician, who cures his patients sometimes, relieves his patients often, and comforts his patients always.... The human person is a truly awesome creation; we are a unified person. To care for a person experiencing illness requires the recognition that...they are not only affected in a physical manner, but also psychologically, emotionally, and spiritually.... Dr. Fenske recognizes that patient-centered care...is uniquely possible when he, as a physician, lives out his faith, rather than hides it.... Dr. Fenske also urges physicians to act by stating: 'Flying under the radar isn't an option. So, rather than allowing ourselves to be bullied into silent submission by those who reject Christ, we need to stand firm and be obedient to the One to whom we must all give account....' This is not an easy message, but he reminds us of the awesome creation that is truly explained when we recognize that we are the creature and we are not God."

- **Alex Schadenberg,** Executive Director, Euthanasia Prevention Coalition

"Dr. Ted Fenske's new book could not have come at a better time. Many in medicine feel they are being asked to choose between their faith and their jobs. Dr. Fenske's book makes a compelling case for how to be a faithful doctor in difficult times."

- **Stephanie Fennelly**, Executive Director, The Wilberforce Project

"The heartbeat of our ministry is to help Christians be effective ambassadors for Christ in everyday conversations. This doesn't mean that every conversation has to be directly about Jesus, but it does mean we want Christians to have a tone and demeanor that always points back to Christ. As I read Dr. Fenske's great resource for Christian medical staff, I was blessed to see him model this approach.... I appreciated the many examples he gave of thoughtful questions he asked patients about their spiritual experiences.... If you work in the medical community, whether you are a believer of Christ or not, I encourage you to pick up *Keeping Faith in Medicine*. It is a great template for how you can be both a good doctor and a good servant."
- **Jojo Ruba,** Executive Director, Faith Beyond Belief Ministries

"*Keeping Faith in Medicine* is a prophetic call to doctors who are believers to become *Christian physicians*. It is also a witness to the medical community of a higher purpose and calling, filled with compassion and truth that point to eternal realities. It is imperative we practise the clear instruction in this book if we are to pass on a living faith that will transform medicine and bring true healing to our patients in life and death. Ted takes the reader on a very personal and honest journey as he recounts hard lessons learned and faith reborn by the sovereign grace of God. I encourage all who read this book to enter the transformative life and calling of physician in service of the one true Healer, Jehovah Rapha."
- **Blaine Achen,** MD, FRCPC, Assistant Clinical Professor, Department of Anesthesiology & Pain Medicine, University of Alberta, Cardiac Anaesthesia

Published by Ezra Press, a ministry of the Ezra Institute for
Contemporary Christianity

PO Box 9, Stn. Main.
Grimsby, ON
L3M 1M0.

Unless otherwise noted, Scripture quotations are taken from the New
International Version. Copyright 1973, 1978, 1984, 2011 Biblica.

Cover design by Barbara Vasconcelos
Interior design and illustrations by Rachel Eras

For volume pricing please contact the Ezra Institute:
info@ezrainstitute.ca

Keeping Faith in Medicine: Navigating Secularized Healthcare with
Grace and Truth
ISBN: 978-1-989169-07-0

Dedicated to the students of the Christian Medical/Dental Association and the Federation of Christian Nurses, who have been an encouragement to me and inspired this work.

"Be on your guard; stand firm in the faith; be courageous; be strong. Do everything in love."
1 Cor. 16:13-14

TABLE OF CONTENTS

ACKNOWLEDGEMENTS

In the fall of 2007, my wife, Tanya, and I began inviting students from the Christian Medical/Dental Association to our home for monthly gatherings of fellowship, worship, and discussion. Through this ministry of hospitality and nurture, I learned all the more how the secularized world of healthcare is hard on believers, and that Christian students and healthcare professionals alike need encouragement to live out their faith, as well as biblical equipping to understand how best that can be done. This book is very much a product of those meetings. I am indebted to these students of medicine, dentistry, and nursing who have kept me accountable to my practice of medicine as a priestly calling. It is for Christian healthcare students, first and foremost, that I felt compelled to write this manuscript, which I hope will be of service to them in their careers ahead, as they practice in the presence of God.

With a subject material of this scope, developed over an entire career, it can be a daunting task to know where to begin with thanks and acknowledgements. By God's grace, this isn't my predicament. He has given me a wonderfully supportive wife to do life with, including writing this book. Like Bond relies on Q, McCoy leans on Spock, and peanut butter needs jelly, Tanya has been my secret weapon, voice of calm in storms, and added sweetness. She has been my trusty backboard off of which I have bounced ideas over the years, and has offered significant behind-the-scenes shaping and editing of this manuscript from its earliest of forms. I want to thank her for making it possible for me to have the protected time to tackle this project, which has brought me closer in my walk with the Lord, and given me a fuller sense of how to keep my faith central in my practice of medicine.

The Christian faith communities that I've been part of over the years have each played an important role in my spiritual growth and faith development. The holy community at St. John the Evangelist Anglican Church in Edmonton, has been particularly instrumental. There I have experienced intimate fellowship, gained increased respect for church tradition, learned the value of the sacraments, and been guided into a life of prayer. The list of saints is a lengthy one and includes Rev. Don Aellen, who instructed me in the way of our church fathers, Rev. Mary Charlotte Wilcox, who introduced me to prayer ministry and made the gospel attractive, Norman Sieweke, who gave me a heart for worship, Dr. Mark Peppler, who unpacked Scripture with me in our early morning Bible studies, and Dr. Mark Belletrutti, who fanned into flame the idea of this book when it was but a glimmer. I would also like to thank Pastor Jason Hagen, from Fellowship Baptist Church, Edmonton, whose enduring wise words and bold witness, during these hostile times, have been a welcome inspiration, convicting me, encouraging me, and bolstering me to live out my faith fully and unashamedly.

Having Christian role models in the medical profession has been most helpful for the development of this book. I would like to acknowledge and thank my colleagues from the Christian Medical/Dental Association (CMDA) for being a much needed community of professional support and encouragement. In particular, I would like to thank Dr. John Patrick for consistently articulating a reasonable faith, and for prodding me to live a life worthy of this priestly calling. The local CMDA chapter meetings and National Conferences have given me insight into the contemporary challenges that face Christian healthcare professionals, and provided some of the tools needed to develop a winsome defense of the faith. I would like to acknowledge and thank Larry Worthen and Stephanie Potter from the CMDA National Office, for their tireless leadership and organizational work, and for inviting me to contribute to FOCUS Magazine, which has given me the opportunity to develop some of this book's content. I would also like to thank Dr. Dan Reilly for his careful review of the manuscript and useful editorial comments, and Dr. Margaret Cottle for her helpful scrutiny of the text and general encouragement. In addition, I would like to give due credit to my prayer partners, Dr. Terrence McQuiston, for his thoughtful insights and encouraging friendship provided over our Saturday morning Skype sessions, and Dr. Tom Noga, for emanating such a deep love of the Lord during our discussions of Scripture, shared over mid-week mugs of London fog.

I owe a special thanks to Stephanie Gray, the founder of the prolife ministry, *Love Unleashes Life*, for her gracious review of the manuscript. Her detailed and discerning suggestions were particularly helpful in the final stages of the writing.

Finally, I would like to express deep gratitude for the leadership and faculty of the Ezra Institute of Contemporary Christianity (EICC). In particular, I want to thank Rev. Joseph Boot, founder of the Institute, for his warm friendship, wise mentorship, and for encouraging me to express why I still believe. His provocative call to redeem all spheres of culture under Christ's lordship inspired this book, and his clarification of how my faith in Jesus acts as the necessary precondition for my medical practice provided its needed epistemological foundation. As well, I want to thank my friend (and ski buddy) Randall Currie, for his tireless work in establishing EICC, and for gently steering me in the direction of Reformational thought, and keeping me accountable to Kingdom work. In addition, I am indebted to Ryan Eras, the Director of Content and Publishing at the Ezra Institute, for his penetrating editorial comments, his eye for detail, and his faithful commitment to bring this work to timely completion.

Soli Deo Gloria

FOREWORD

DR. JOHN PATRICK, M.B., B.S., M.R.C.P., M.D

It is a great pleasure to be asked to write this foreword. One of the great joys of our Lord's way of teaching us discipleship is that he asks us to be simply obedient in little things without much detail about how it will work out en route. But with small acts of obedience come hints and intimations of a future beyond imagination. In a lonely world we find ourselves constantly running in to brothers and sisters in the Lord. Such was the case, when the grace of God introduced me to Dr. Fenske.

All of us at times can get into the "Elijah Syndrome" of "I only I am left." Of course, it is not and will never be true. This book is difficult to categorize; it has elements of a biography but also of an intellectual and a spiritual journey from a Christian home to medical school, with the almost-universal departure from active faith, and then the prodigal's return. But this prodigal has told the story with warts and all and the result bristles with authenticity.

The modern world is leaving the church out of its life because it sees the church as inauthentic, indeed hypocritical, and it is a largely valid judgment. How many of us as doctors (and this is a book primarily for doctors) have gone to church after a very bad week only to be confronted with a service which is almost banal in its failure to speak into our hearts about the existential pain we call life. But that is not the case here. The rubber hits the road in ways which most doctors will immediately recognize in their own experience but also in a way that challenges of our usual failure to learn from our sins. Confession is not common – real confession as in the case of Isaiah in the temple.

However, Dr. Fenske doesn't leave us with the existential pain endured and then locked in a filing cabinet of the soul but tells of his own renewal through suffering. It is a recurrent phenomenon in a Christian life. What is at stake here is to understand that there is no gift from God, which he does not usually remove, not permanently but only to remove the evil sense of entitlement which we have attached to it, then returning it as a gift to be used to introduce others to the giver. (Adapted from Fenelon) Romans 5 lays it out as a sequence; suffering is given to lead to endurance to character to hope based on the love we have received from God.

Not everyone will be comfortable as Dr. Fenske lays out the ways in which he bears witness to colleagues and patients. I suspect most of you will be challenged by the discipline with which he goes about practicing the means of grace, but there is no doubt that it is time to awake from our slumber and start to be not only able but also to actually give reasons for our faith winsomely. This book will help.

JOHN PATRICK holds M.B., B.S., M.R.C.P. and M.D. degrees from the University of London and St. George's Hospital Medical School in London, and is a British trained biochemist who was a former Professor of Clinical Nutrition in the Department of Biochemistry and Pediatrics at the University of Ottawa, and is currently the President and Professor of the History of Science, Medicine and Faith at Augustine College, and long-member and leader in CMDA Canada.

Sydenham's Oath

Thomas Sydenham (1624 – 1689)

"It becomes every person who purposes to give himself to the care of others, seriously to consider the four following things: First, that he must one day give account to the Supreme Judge of all the lives entrusted to his care. Second, that all his skill and knowledge and energy, as they have been given him by God, so they should be exercised for His glory and the good of mankind, and not for mere gain or ambition. Third, and not more beautifully than truly, let him reflect that he has undertaken the care of no mean creature; for, in order that he may estimate the value, the greatness of the human race, the only begotten Son of God became Himself a man, and thus ennobled it with His divine dignity, and far more than this, died to redeem it. And fourth, that the doctor being himself a mortal human being, should be diligent and tender in relieving his suffering patients, inasmuch as he himself must one day be a like sufferer."

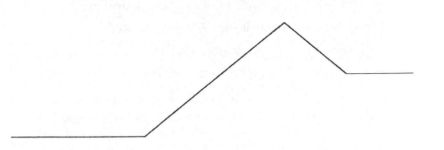

INTRODUCTION

"For I am not ashamed of the gospel, because it is the power of God
that brings salvation to everyone who believes."

Romans 1:16

THE PRIESTLY CALLING OF MEDICINE

A few questions might come to mind on glancing at this book title,
such as "What's a heart specialist writing about *faith in medicine* for?"
And while hopefully not, "Medicine is based on science; so, who needs
faith?!" other questions might be, "How can we as Christian healthcare

professionals live out our faith in this contemporary, and increasingly anti-Christian climate of medicine?" Or even, "Shouldn't we just remain under the radar and keep our Christian beliefs a private matter?" Since I've been asking myself the first question quite a bit of recent, I'll tackle it straight off and then address the others along with some general comments about the structure of this book and my hopes for how it might be helpful.

I work as a clinical cardiologist in a tertiary-care hospital in downtown Edmonton managing patients with heart diseases of every sort. Although the demands of my practice consume much of my time, I consider myself, first and foremost, a follower of Christ, and liken my role in the hospital to that of a *sheep in wolf's clothing*. Donning my white lab coat and stethoscope *mantle* with ID lanyard, I gain ready access to the vast and varied mission field of medicine with unlimited opportunities to shine God's light. While I've dog-eared the pages of Harrison's and Braunwald textbooks aplenty and added margin notes and yellow highlighting as proof, it's my beat-up NIV which most informs my practice, and my personal faith in Christ its focus. The list of letters that follow my name, which loosely translate as, *went to school for a long time*, were hard-earned and have served me well in my frontline clinical work. Nonetheless, I join the apostle Paul in considering "them a loss compared to the surpassing greatness of knowing Christ Jesus my Lord, for whose sake I have lost all things. I consider them rubbish that I may gain Christ" (Phil. 3:8-9).

I hadn't always planned on a career in medicine – I had much higher aspirations. "I wanna be like you when I grow up, Daddy," I remember saying as I climbed onto my father's lap to show him my artwork from school. It was a smudged crayon drawing depicting two black-robed figures (the bigger one representing my father and the smaller one, me) with a multi-colored scribble of a stained-glass window as a backdrop.

Although I didn't know exactly what a Navy Chaplain did, I knew it was a pretty important job – and just as important as the firemen and astronauts that my friends had drawn for our class assignment. I saw this firsthand when I visited him on the Stadacona Base. Uniformed soldiers would freeze to attention as he walked past, and even the higher-ranking officers would stand and salute him. And when my father spoke, the room would quiet and people would listen. Even though I didn't understand all of what my dad preached about, I'd regularly skip out of Sunday school class so I could listen to him. And though I found it kind of embarrassing when he would raise his voice into the higher decibel ranges or slam his fist on the pulpit, I knew he was saying something significant. He packed out the pews, and I later learned how he had changed countless lives. I witnessed some of this, as well. We'd often have reformed alcoholics over from the base for lunch – real hairy-knuckle types – who would gently give witness to Dad's ministry of reconciliation in their broken lives. Needless to say, I was very proud of him. So, to further prove to everyone within earshot my intentions to follow in his footsteps, I'd regularly clomp around the hardwood floors of our home as a young child in my father's relatively boat-sized shoes.

My vocational plans took further shape when our family was invited to listen to a special guest speaker at a local church – Dr. Robert McClure, a medical missionary and past Moderator of the United Church of Canada. Being a pastor's family, we were given honorary seats in the front pew of the filled-to-capacity church, while others had to sit in the basement and listen to the sermon piped-in. As an eleven-year old, I shivered with excitement as he described his exotic travels and medical trials. And then things got personal. While Dr. McClure recounted a tense surgical situation in his mission hospital in China, and about how he had to send a young boy to urgently fetch a particular instrument so he could complete an emergency procedure, he paused for a moment and pointed directly at me. "Just like this boy, here," he said, as all eyes turned to my reddening face. Instantly, I was famous (at least for the duration of the coffee hour that day). When I was later introduced to him during coffee time, he shook my hand, ruffled my hair, and asked if I'd thought about becoming a doctor and doing medical missions, too. Well, of course I hadn't. But from that time on, the prospect dug deep into my imagination. Dr. McClure opened up my world that day to consider what Christian ministry could look like beyond the pulpit. By describing the provision of medical care as a calling from God – to be *His* hands and *His* feet in alleviating suffering and promoting healing – he gave me an early glimpse into the priestly role of the healthcare provider.

My understanding of this priestly role was further developed on my first day of medical school with the Dean of Medicine's welcoming address. He opened with the wise words of Edward Trudeau – the founder of the tuberculosis sanitarium – who said, "The role of the physician is to cure sometimes, to relieve often, and to comfort always." This enduring adage speaks to the comprehensive scope of healing, as being both physical and spiritual in nature. From an etymology standpoint, this broader definition of healing makes a certain amount of sense. The words *health*, *wholeness*, and *holiness* all share the same Old English root, *hal*, which means 'whole'. Similarly, the Latin word, *salvation*, is derived from *salve*, the commonly used synonym for ointment, and has at its root the word *health* and the implication, *total restoration*.[1] Paracelsus, the acclaimed physician of antiquity, held that diseases originate in the realm of nature, but healing comes from the realm of the spirit. In line with this, I've come to appreciate that there is a remarkable overlap between the practice of medicine and the work of the Christian pastor. Remuneration aside, both vocations have to do with providing care and seeking remedy to human suffering. In a like manner, the confidential

4

communication between doctor and patient mirrors, to a similar extent, the honoured trust between pastor and parishioner. Both forms of communication are not only privileged, but are undertaken in the search of healing, wholeness and, ultimately, of salvation. I'm sometimes taken aback by just how much my clinic feels like a confessional (minus the privacy screen and kneelers, of course). Within short minutes of our time together, and with little prompting, patients share with me very intimate details of their lives, seeking a sympathetic ear and earnest counsel. Such tender moments remind me of my privileged role in medicine and reinforce my conviction that it is a priestly calling.

In our contemporary cultural climate, however, the suggestion that the practice of medicine is a priestly calling isn't a popular one and, in fact, is very much opposed. I recall being told repeatedly during my training years by my superiors that the medical practitioner must dissociate their own personal values from their medical obligations. We were admonished not to permit our particular beliefs to enter the hallowed halls of medicine lest we usher in elements of bias that would hinder our abilities to provide patient-centered care. The stark truth that the Christian worldview alone makes sense of patient-centered care, and provides the foundation for putting it into practice, was a foreign notion to them. For the populist purveyors of medical education, the acceptable approach for Christian healthcare providers is to keep their beliefs a strictly private matter; safely hidden away, leaving the instructors' divinized naturalism unchallenged. Of course, a faith that can be boxed up neat n' tidy isn't much alive in the first place. As G.K. Chesterton pointed out, "A dead thing can go with the stream, but only a living thing can go against it." If being a Christian is merely trying to be a nice person on weekdays and attending church in the suburbs some Sundays, what's its value? As Jesus cautioned, "You are the salt of the earth. But if the salt loses its saltiness, how can it be made salty again? It is no longer good for anything, except to be thrown out and trampled underfoot" (Matt. 5:13). We are called to proclaim the gospel and preserve the Christian heritage of our culture, and that means having a certain visibility. Flying under the radar isn't an option. So, rather than allowing ourselves to be bullied into silent submission by those who reject Christ, we need to stand firm and be obedient to the One to whom we must all give account, knowing that where there is judgement, there is also salvation.

"Easier said than done," one might counter. And I would agree; the *How To* part of faith application can be challenging. The secular terrain of medicine may prove difficult trekking, but navigation is still possible. As Chesterton also said, "The Christian ideal has not been tried and found wanting. It has been found difficult; and left untried." To try it successfully, we need to be clear about what we believe and, in particular, the fundamentals of our faith – the plain, straight-up gospel message. A glance back at one of the most storied periods in NFL history might illustrate this point. It's said of Vince Lombardi, legendary coach for the Green Bay Packers, that he would begin training camp with a most elemental statement. "Gentlemen," he would say to the seasoned players as he held up a pigskin in full view, "this is a football."[2] And although some of the gathered players may have scoffed or smirked at the obvious statement, Lombardi wanted to stress an appreciation of the basics. To effectively live out our Christian faith in hostile times, it's critical that we also ingrain in our minds such a similarly elemental view of the gospel. As Lombardi aptly proved by taking his struggling Wisconsin team to five world championships, keeping focused on the fundamentals can make all the difference. Without appreciating the overview foundation, knowing the details can sometimes be of little value. But *with* such grounding, even small gains can add up to something quite significant and more than we can ask or imagine.

To provide an analogous *this-is-a-football* visual for the gospel fun-

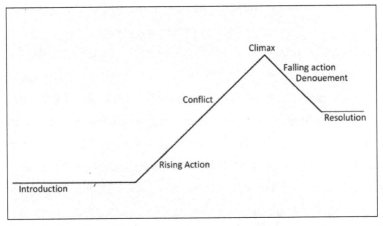

Figure 1. Short Story Plotline

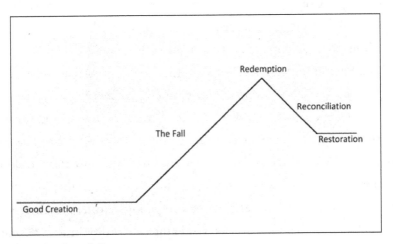

Figure 2. Gospel Contour

damentals, I make use of a simplified schematic representation of the biblical narrative, which follows the short-story plotline (Fig. 1). As you might recall from grade school English class, the plotline scaffolding begins with a short horizontal segment representing the introduction of the story. The line then slopes upwards signifying the rising action or conflict in the story, followed by a downward line denoting the falling action or denouement. The apex or plateau of the two adjoining lines represents the turning point or climax of the story. And finally, the resolution of the story is indicated by a return to the horizontal baseline.

By assigning the key biblical features that comprise the gospel message in its fullness to each of the five contour elements of the short story plotline, I develop what I refer to as the Gospel Contour (Fig. 2). Such conceptualization can help us guard against accepting a truncated view of the gospel, which reduces its application to some compartmentalized area of our lives, rather than every sphere. While I've never tried using this Gospel Contour schema in a locker room setting, in PowerPoint presentations to medical students it works pretty well.

The Gospel Contour, with its allocated features of the biblical narrative, forms the structural layout of this book and acts as the general outline for discussions around Christian engagement with the medical sphere. Each chapter is devoted to one of the five contour features and begins with a brief summary of its contained narrative. While I recognize that the summary may seem a review, I think it's important to clearly state the basics (It was a winning strategy for Vince, after all). After the summary preface, I describe the competing cultural narratives and the difficulties that arise from considering our reality in this manner. Addressing each of the five narrative elements in turn, I contrast them to the prevailing cultural worldviews that we come into contact with in the practice of medicine. I then discuss how we can lean on the gospel, not only to guard ourselves from getting sidetracked into ungodly thinking,

8

but also to more effectively be salt and light for the patients under our care. To illustrate some of the difficulties that can arise when a non-biblical worldview is adopted in medical practice, I share some of my own faith struggles that I've had over the years. Then to provide a means of protection from adopting an impoverished worldview, I present various practical spiritual disciplines which I have incorporated into my routine to help keep my medical practice God-focussed. Using illustrative patient encounters, I then detail how we might engage competing cultural storylines with the gospel truth in the clinical setting. For ease of memory and review, each chapter concludes with a bulleted summary of the key points from the section, followed by a series of questions for personal reflection or group discussion

We practice medicine in biblically hostile times. Although Christianity is still considered the largest world religion, comprising nearly a third of the earth's population, there has been a sharp decline in Christian church affiliation over the last number of decades, and a simultaneous upsurge in secularization.[3] This decline of the Christian influence in our society has had serious consequences for healthcare provision. The value of human life has been put into question and is no longer considered sanctified. Family planning and maternal health have become synonymous with abortion provision. With over 100,000 pre-born killed every year in Canada, and no laws to protect them, the womb now represents the least safe space for a baby to take refuge. The decriminalization and simultaneous embrace of physician-assisted suicide has irreparably marred the doctor/patient relationship and placed healthcare providers in the untenable position of having to negotiate between suicide prevention and suicide promotion. As a result of our new laws, palliative care has become confused with suicide assistance, and vulnerable populations, including the elderly and disabled, have been placed in mortal danger. The sexualization of our culture and widespread endorsement of gender discordance has resulted in medical therapies and surgical interventions that are diametrically opposed to human flourishing and creational design. Conscience rights for healthcare providers have become subordinated to unchallenged patient autonomy, and the priestly role of medicine has been reduced to one of technical provider. In brief, this current era represents a time of unparalleled challenge for the Christian healthcare provider.

The present challenges, although daunting, bring with them opportunities for us to be salt and light. As Martin Luther said, "Where the battle rages, there the loyalty of the soldier is proved." To be loyal to King Jesus, we need to be prepared to address the hot-button issues of our day, particularly as they intersect with healthcare provision, and provide resistance and push back as need be. In this applied survey of the gospel, I have not shied away from difficult areas nor considered any topic taboo. Using clinical examples, I have attempted to illustrate how we might negotiate the challenging areas of LGBT medicine, physician assisted suicide, pornography addiction, and medical futility, and do so with grace and truth.

As Christian healthcare providers, we need encouragement to live out our faith, and role-modelling to understand how that can be done. My intention is that this book will provide both some practical equipping for Christian healthcare professionals to aptly identify and more confidently address gospel opportunities as they arise in clinical practice, as well as provide some level of encouragement for practitioners to embrace their priestly role, whether as a doctor, nurse, pharmacist, dentist or a provider from one of the equally valuable allied healthcare disciplines. As we accept the gauntlet laid before us, we would do well to keep the words of the apostle Paul in our minds when he said, "Be on your guard; stand firm in the faith; be courageous; be strong. Do everything in love" (1 Cor. 16:13-14).

CHAPTER NOTES

1. Joe Boot. "Health, Salvation and the Kingdom of God." *Jubilee*. Spring 2012.
2. David Maraniss. *When Pride Still Mattered: A Life Of Vince Lombardi*. Simon & Schuster. 2000.
3. *The Changing Global Religious Landscape*. Pew Research Centre. April 5, 2017.

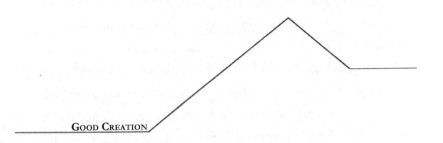

CHAPTER 1

IDENTITY CRISIS AND CONFUSION

"I praise you because I am fearfully and wonderfully made; your works
are wonderful, I know that full well."

Psalm 139:14

IDENTITY AS A CREATIONAL ISSUE

Beginning with the beginning, the first feature of the gospel narrative
is the *Good Creation*. Placed on the initial horizontal segment of the
short-story plotline, this portion of the biblical contour embodies
the explanation of our origins, and represents the foundation for our

self-understanding. The Creation account poetically details the cosmic formation of the universe culminating with the bringing into being of mankind – God's opus magnum. When God said, "Let us make man in our image, in our likeness" (Gen. 1:26), we were given the privileged position as the centerpiece of it all. The creation doctrine of Imago Dei refers to the imprint that God has placed on the human soul, and provides the biblical explanation for our unique attributes, such as reasoning and our sense of morality. It is because we are created in God's image that we, too, can create, design, and craft, as well as communicate with spoken and written language, demonstrate covenantal love, and express ourselves in praise and worship. In brief, this sacred imprint is what renders human life precious. As a result of this designation, we are unlike all other created beings. Named His children, we have been titled as image bearers in order that we might represent God to the rest of creation. And since God's daily work of preserving and governing the world is inseparable from His act of calling the cosmos into being, this first segment of the gospel contour also represents God's providential and sovereign governance of the universe, including His active and intimate involvement in the details of our daily lives.

Our medical culture outright rejects the gospel narrative of Creation. Reducing it to mere myth or ancient allegory, contemporary medicine has joined the chorus of secular culture and embraced the theory of evolution as the prevailing explanation for the origin of the universe. Denying the created order that "God has made plain" (Rom. 1:19), medical elites expound the narrative that undirected natural processes are responsible for all aspects of our material reality. Driven by random chance, and enabled by the magic wand of time, the story of evolution renders providence and prophecy unnecessary. If God is allowed to retain any role at all, it's limited to that of a deistic *first mover* player. Domesticated in this way, God is no longer sovereign, and has only indirect

16

involvement in the outworking of the universe. Of course, if God is removed entirely from the origins equation, so too is our image-of-God identity. In this way, rejection of the biblical narrative necessitates the abandonment of our divine imprint. As a result, human beings are no longer considered "a little lower than the angels; crowned with glory and honor" (Ps. 8:5), but rather thought to be evolved from primordial muck, and on par with all other living beings. In this common-ancestor view of life on earth, people are regarded as being no different than animals, just temporarily occupying a higher rung on the evolutionary ladder. As such, human beings are lowered in their value, and plants and animals are elevated. As animal rights activist, Ingrid Newkirk said, "A rat is a pig is a dog is a boy. They are all animals." Taken to an even further extreme, this same sentiment asserts that "Whales are people, too!"[1] In this contemporary cultural narrative, we are no longer considered created in God's image, but tasked to create our own image and fashion our own identity. In other words, if God is not our maker, than we are left to pick up the slack and do our own making. The American artist Bobbie Carlyle visually expressed this perspective with her provocative bronze sculpture of a male figure chiselling himself out of the rocks entitled, *Self-Made Man*. Depicted this way, our identity is something we can continually invent and reinvent, as best suits our present circumstances. Characterised by mantras like, "be true to yourself" and "I did it my way," our prevailing cultural narrative holds tightly to a radical individualism. Standing in stark contrast to a self-denying and God-directed biblical identity, a secular identity is a solo project, and is sought by self-focussed plans and inwardly directed labours.

The practical difficulty with a self-made identity is that it simply doesn't deliver. No matter how many times we try to invent or re-invent ourselves, our core needs for acceptance, significance and security remain unmet. This is particularly the case when disease and death come knocking. A fabricated identity will wear thin when applied to the trials of the world, and come undone when challenged by serious illness. Efforts to be accepted on our own terms will do little to dispel the deep-seated feelings of loneliness and abandonment, which only become magnified when we're sick in bed. Attempts to blow our own horn and construct a personal significance through work or achievements merely confirms a low self-esteem, and becomes quickly stripped away by an open-at-the-back, one-size-fits-nobody hospital gown. Despite our best efforts to develop security by building a net worth of stocks and bonds, anxieties for the future remain and fears continue to haunt, especially when disability claims fail to cover the mounting bills. When faced with the spectre of illness and disease, a non-biblical self-understanding can easily lead to identity crisis and confusion.

MISPLACED IDENTITY MEETS MISFORTUNE

In the past, I've made the mistake of attempting to understand my identity outside of God's definition. Even though I generally accepted the biblical narrative of creation and believed that I was created in God's image, I allowed myself to get swept along with a secular formulation of my identity. Being in the world distracted me from not being of the world, and despite knowing better, I've repeatedly gravitated towards placing my identity onto things other than Christ. In grade school, for example, it was all about my grades. As I negotiated those awkward teen years, I allowed my academic accolades to define my core self-understanding. When I hit university, this self-understanding took on an obsessive dimension. In my harried pre-med study years, I allowed my studies to consume me. As I burned the midnight oil memorizing biochemistry formulas, I sweated for the praise of my professors and sacrificed my young-adult years on the altar of the *Grade Point Aver-*

age. My general disposition and demeanor would rise or fall depending upon how high or low my posted marks were on the lecture room door. This performance-based identity continued through my medical school years and residency training, and steered me further and further from a Christ-based understanding of myself.

In the realm of medicine, it's easy to get sucked into the vortex of worldly thinking, including the way we think about our identity. I was certainly no exception, particularly in my first few stressful years of practice. As a young staff cardiologist, my identity was very much anchored to my profession. Consistent with our medical culture, which emphasizes a work-based identity, I defined myself by what I did. At social gatherings, for example, I would first introduce myself with my professional involvement. I talked shop over meals and even linked my family vacations to conferences away. My peers did the same, so it seemed normal to me. I had a young needy family at that time, new financial pressures of overhead and mortgage, and heavy hospital responsibilities – managing the coronary care unit, covering ward consultations by day and taking emergency calls through the night. So, to better establish my fledgling practice and prove my mettle to my colleagues, I buried myself in my work. With my neglected Bible collecting dust next to the Encyclopedia Britannica, I then allowed my Scripture reading and church attendance to slide. "I just need some down time, Honey!" was how I persuaded my wife to let me stay at home Sunday mornings in my pyjamas and catch up on my paperwork pile, while she and the boys went to worship. It certainly felt like I was running on empty with no time to waste. So, when I did get a reprieve from my hospital commitments, I was reluctant to spend my time sitting on a hard pew and listening to a hand-bell ensemble version of *Shine Jesus Shine*, when I could be whittling down my burgeoning to-do list. But as a result of not being rooted and established in a church family, my understanding of who I was, and who I figured God must be, began to shift. It was almost imperceptible at first, but little by little my thinking became more secularized and my understanding of who I was in Christ diminished.

Without being surrounded by the support, encouragement, and accountability of a Christian community, my faith commitments began to erode, one by one, and slowly became nominalized. Instead of having Holy Scripture inform my thoughts, my thinking became shaped to conform to the world's ways. Faced with a problem, I'd approach its answer from a worldly perspective, leaning on my own understanding, and not on the Lord's. In terms of personal significance, for example, I looked everywhere except to the one true source of self-worth, our Heavenly Father. Caught up in career building, I began to believe that my true value came from *what I did*, rather than from *what God has done* for me. Disregarding the apostle Paul's declaration that I am significant because I have God's Holy Spirit dwelling within me (1 Cor. 3:16), I allowed the world's view of significance to dominate my thinking and behaviours. I figured that the more letters I strung behind my name, and the thicker I padded my curriculum vitae, and longer I stretched out my list of publications, the more significant I'd become. It's a soul-sucking view of significance, and one that Timothy Keller cautioned against by saying, "When work is your identity, if you're successful it goes to your head, and if you're a failure it goes to your heart."[2]

When it came to my need for acceptance, I chose the popular path of people pleaser. In our cardiology group, for example, I was considered the *Yes Man*. Being always able to say "Sure, I can do it" to the black hole of hospital work was how I came to define myself. If there were left-over consults accumulated in the emergency room to be seen, I'd see them. If a colleague needed a call night covered, I'd cover it. And if there was a last-minute consult request, I'd tack it onto my urgent waitlist. "Gonna be home late again, Sweetheart" was the refrain my wife became accustomed to hearing. When challenges arose, I met them with an affirmative nod of my head, and buckled down and worked all the harder. I bought into the pervasive lie that "God helps those who help themselves," and forgot the truth that God accepts me because I am His child (John 1:12). I believed that my acceptance came from working hard and receiving kudos from others, and completely disregarded Paul's caution that "If I were still trying to please people, I would not be a servant of Christ" (Gal. 1:10).

In reference to my need for security, I did what any self-respecting cardiologist would do faced with financial strain: I jumped on the monetary bandwagon and accumulated more wealth. While mocking the bumper sticker slogan, "He who dies with the most toys wins," I would, nonetheless, fall in line at the box stores on Sunday myself. In so doing, I not only broke the Fourth Commandment by desecrating the Sabbath, I reduced my image-bearing identity to the base level of petty purchaser. Over time, I began to believe that my security depended upon my financial statements. It made a certain amount of sense to me at the time – the more billings I could generate, the more savings I would accrue; and the more stocks and bonds I could stockpile, the more security I would assure. Where my treasure was, so my heart was also (Matt. 6:21). Far from my thoughts was the fact that I was already a citizen of Heaven (Phil. 3:20). No, my security had to be wrought in the here and now, by me being in control, taking, grasping, clutching.... and trying to buy my stairway to Heaven. So, like the parable of the rich fool, I attempted to store up riches for myself, but I wasn't rich towards God (Luke 12:16-21).

I didn't realize just how impoverished my identity had become until it was challenged by illness, and found wanting. Although it occurred many years ago, I recall it like yesterday. I had taken the afternoon off work early to enjoy the last of the summer sun with my family at the park. I was enjoying a game of tag with my boys and running from the monkey bars to the slide. Then, as if struck by lightning on a cloudless day, I collapsed face down on the sand. As I lay there bewildered, I found myself entering into a thick haze that was getting hazier. It was like when you awaken from a deep afternoon nap and you don't remember who you are or where, and you just lie there perplexed with a drool bridge connecting your mouth to the pillow. My confusion intensified when my wife, horrified to see me limping towards her with drooping face, announced that she was calling the ambulance because I was having a stroke.

"Having a what?" I tried to say, but my mouth moved like I'd just come out of the dentist chair post root canal. "Are you crazy?" I tried to argue. "How could I be having a stroke? I'm just 41 years old and in perfect health! And besides, I'm the medical doctor here, and this is not a stroke. I've simply... uh... bumped my funny bone... and once the funny part wears off... I'll be fine. Let's just wait it out. Don't call the ambulance. It'll just frighten the boys," I pleaded.

But she would have none of it. With a determined look on her face, she sat me down, supported my back with one arm, and promptly dialled 911. In the blink of an eye, I was no longer the doctor responding to a medical crisis, but a patient in the throes of one.

Within the hour, I was diagnosed with a carotid artery dissection. It resulted in a dense right middle cerebral artery thrombotic stroke involving an extensive area of my brain. Unlike the majority of cases with a similar diagnosis, I survived. Thanks to the timely state-of-the-art treatments that I received in the form of thrombolytic therapy and bare metal stenting, my physical recovery was nothing short of a miracle. I not only recovered use of my left side, I was able to walk within three days, and released from hospital in a week. Nonetheless, returning to work was more problematic than I had anticipated. Since I didn't walk with a limp, could move both my limbs, and was able to smile without making a snarl, I figured that I would be able to return to the *bridge* and proceed "full-steam ahead, Captain." But as soon as my work day entered into *warp factor one*, I was finished. I couldn't keep up, think fast enough, or even begin to multitask. If there was the least interruption in my sleep, I was unable to make a cup of coffee, let alone float a Swan-Ganz catheter. I had survived the stroke, but my ability to work hadn't, and my work-based identity was unable to make sense of the quandary. Questions flooded my mind. If I was unable to work full-time, particularly with all the same overhead expenses, "What kind of security could I expect?" Unable to complete my research project, publish my papers, or proceed with my academic credentialing, "Where would I go for significance?" And if I could no longer take night-call, manage the CCU, or cover emergency consultation, "How could I be accepted by my cardiology peers?" In brief, "If I can't work as a fully-functioning cardiologist, then who am I?"

These questions betrayed my misplaced identity. The existential suffering that I experienced following my stroke could have been prevented, or at least diminished, had I taken better care of protecting my identity in Christ. At its center, our identity is not only a cultural issue, but a creational one that needs to be defined by our Creator. Our core identity doesn't reside in our domain to create and recreate, but rather is contained within the eternal relationship of the triune living God. By necessity, our *I am* needs to be grounded in the *Great I am*. As detailed by Neil Anderson, when we fail to grasp this biblical reality, choosing instead something smaller or distorted, we generate within ourselves an unquenchable thirst for personal significance, social acceptance, and individual security.[3]

So, rather than looking inwards to understand our identity, we need to look beyond ourselves and be open to receive the transcendent words that "The Lord your God is with you, he is mighty to save. He will take great delight in you, he will quiet you with his love, he will rejoice over you with singing" (Zeph. 3:17). Our personal identity needs to rest on the foundational understanding that we are children of a loving Heavenly Father, who has counted the number of hairs on our heads, and knows our thoughts before we speak them. We are not the accidental by-product of some random chance aberration, but rather are "fearfully and wonderfully made" (Ps. 139:14). God designed and created us, and intimately knows the details of who we are better than we do. Any attempt to meet our core needs outside of a personal relationship with Christ will be met with frustration and futility.

PROTECTING OUR BIBLICAL IDENTITY

Since the worldly formulations of identity can't meet our central needs, it's important to foster and protect an identity in Christ, which can. The primary means to nurture such an identity is through a personal relationship with the risen Lord; and the fundamental means to guard an identity in Christ, is by reading Scripture on a regular basis. The Bible not only provides us with a foundational understanding for perceiving reality, and a moral standard from which to make ethical decisions, it offers us direct and ready access to the voice of Christ. To facilitate hearing this voice, it's important to be familiar with the Bible. In order to inwardly digest God's truth for our lives, we need to set time aside and carefully read the Word. So, in addition to the corporate reading of Scripture at church on Sundays, daily personal reflection on the Word is critical. And while group Bible study is helpful in developing depth of understanding, it can become dry ground or degenerate into a social group gathering unless we tap into the living spring of God's intimate revelation on a personal level. The Bible is many things – a big book of divine promises, an epic history of God's relationship with humankind, our moral foundation, and worldview starting point – but included in them, and central on the list, is the personal nature of this revelation to each of us. Scripture is "alive and active. Sharper than any double-edged sword, it penetrates even to dividing soul and spirit, joints and marrow; it judges the thoughts and attitudes of the heart" (Heb. 4:12). Unless we become intimately familiar with Christ's voice in Scripture, we will fail to fully appreciate our God-defined identity, and our priestly calling in medicine.

After my stroke, I began to read from the Bible on a daily basis. As I did so, I found my regular day-to-day thoughts turning back towards God. Like the sheep of His pasture who "follow him because they know His voice" (John 10:4), I became more accustomed to hearing his voice, as well. Over time, my identity in Christ replaced my makeshift identity, shaped by the world, the flesh, and the devil. This meant laying down my frustrated attempts of relying on my work to furnish my self-worth, and using Scripture to reframe my understanding of personal significance. Rather than climbing up the career ladder of medicine to find my value, I leaned into the truth that I am His workmanship and the salt of the earth, and the light of the world (Matt. 5:13-14). Instead of endeavouring to achieve the ever-elusive acceptance of my colleagues and peer group, I turned to God who accepts me as His child "and adopted me as His son through Jesus Christ" (Eph. 1:5). In the place of ruminating over my real estate holdings and the volatile stock exchange to define my security, I looked to God's "plans to prosper and not to harm, plans to give hope and a future" (Jer. 29:11) and His assurance that my "citizenship is in heaven" (Phil 3:20).

DONNING THE FULL ARMOUR OF GOD

To continually protect my identity in Christ, I make a point of accessing

Scripture several times a day. My Bible reading typically begins in the wee hours of the morning. This has less to do with personal piety and more because I regularly suffer from early-morning insomnia. Rather than tossing and turning, and hopelessly trying to force myself to sleep, I get out of bed and open my tattered NIV, continuing where I've left off. To settle my stomach and encourage the return to sleep, I combine my reading of Scripture with a small bowl of cereal. Then, after returning to bed, I close my eyes and restrict my slumbering thoughts to the verses I've just read. In this way, I join the Psalmist who writes, "On my bed I remember you; I think of you through the watches of the night" (Ps. 63:6). I've found this routine to be both an effective means to achieve my forty winks, as well as a practical way to reinforce my God-directed identity. Then, when my alarm later rings and my breakfast preparations begin, I continue my reading as part of my morning devotional.

Reading the Word from the written page allows me to more easily visually memorize passage locations within the text, underline key select words, and jot down notes in the margins for future reference. While I prefer this hard-copy format, I also use a Bible phone app to access Scripture during my workday. I've programmed the Verse of the Day notification for 12 noon. In this way, regardless of how frenzied my morning has become, biblical truth enters my day and soothes me, moves me, and keeps me strong. The arrival of these holy words never ceases to surprise me, and act like the comforting hand of a close friend on the shoulder. As well, since I always have ready access to my phone, I can pull out biblical passages during my downtimes and timely share bookmarked verses with patients, as occasions arise. In this way, I don the full armour of God, complete with "the helmet of salvation and the sword of the Spirit, which is the word of God," so I can stand firm against the devil's schemes (Eph. 6:11-17).

VISUAL PROTECTION OF IDENTITY

We live in a visual world, where a picture is not only worth a thousand words, it's taken the place of words. From graphic newsfeeds and viral memes, to intrusive pop-up ads and luring click bait, we are continually bombarded with attention-grabbing imagery. Anything but benign, this mass exposure and consumption of graphic media can distract from our God-given identity. As Christians, we need to be aware of this danger, and not only discipline our roving eyes so as to minimize such distractions, but also take intentional steps to counter this secular pictorial onslaught. To bring the gospel narrative into this graphic landscape, I make use of various visual cues that help me keep Scripture in mind and my identity in Christ protected. As per the Torah encouragement to "Tie them as symbols on your hands and bind them on your foreheads. Write them on the door-frames of your houses and on your gates" (Deut. 6:8-9), I've incorporated a variety of visuals into my home and workspaces that serve to remind me of *whose* I am and what I'm about.

At home, these visual cues have taken the form of variations on Bible décor. While I recognize that this isn't everyone's taste, it's been a useful way for my wife and I to keep certain Scripture verses in mind and defend us from worldly thinking. On my desk, for example, I have a pottery plaque with the words, "For he has rescued us from the dominion of darkness and brought us into the kingdom of the Son he loves, in whom we have redemption, the forgiveness of sins" (Col. 1:13-14). This inscription sits amongst my papers and pens, reminding me during my work that my acceptance comes from God. In our kitchen, affixed to the cookie cupboard door, we have the verse, "For God did not give us a spirit of timidity, but a spirit of power, of love and of self-discipline" (1 Tim. 1:7). Although it probably did little to thwart our boys from sneaking treats, it has served to reinforce to all who enter our kitchen that our security as a family is found in the Lord. As well, over our

27

entranceway door, we have the Scripture, "I can do all things through Christ who gives me strength" (Phil. 4:13), reminding us in our coming and going that we are significant to God.

In addition to these, I have various pieces of art work hanging on the walls of our living areas that serve as scriptural reminders. In my home office, for example, I have a framed print of Warner Sallman's "The Good Shepherd," with Jesus surrounded by sheep, holding a lamb in one arm and a shepherd's staff in the other. It's an image I've treasured from childhood. In Sunday school, I was given a metallic wallet-sized copy of this image, which I've kept ever since. With each casual glance on the wall, the painting brings to mind Psalm 23, and reminds me of Christ's inclusive compassion and care. On the adjoining wall, by contrast, I have a print of Antonio Ciseri's painting entitled, "Ecce Homo." It's a dramatic scene depicting the scourged Jesus before Pontius Pilate and the on-looking crowds during His passion. This image was featured on the menu page of Focus on the Family's worldview series, *The Truth Project* with Dell Tackett. The powerful image brings to mind not only the passion of Christ, but also our need to give witness to His great love that "While we were still sinners, Christ died for us" (Rom. 5:8).

To take visual cues into my workday, I have chosen specific images for my iPhone wallpaper and laptop screen-saver. For my cell phone, I have an engaging Rien Poortvliet drawing of Jesus with His disciples.[4] This way, every time I call or text or look up a drug dosage, I see the face of Christ, encouraging me, and holding me to account. For my laptop, I chose Rembrandt's *Prodigal Son* as my screensaver, which brings to mind this favorite parable from the Gospel of Luke, and reminds me of our heavenly Father's extravagant forgiveness of sin. In addition to these pictorials, I wear a gospel bracelet on my wrist. It's a simple leather strap with two knots bookending a string of coloured beads. The knots signify birth and death, respectively, and each of the beads represent one of the key gospel features – creation, the fall, redemption, forgiveness, reconciliation, and eternal life. When people at work ask me about the beads, I describe it as my *identification bracelet*. Worn next to my watch, the beaded strap brings the gospel contour to mind and serves as a visual reminder that God alone meets my core needs.

HOLY COMMUNITY PROTECTION OF IDENTITY

Maintaining an identity in Christ is a tall order to fill on one's own. There's a cacophony of competing voices wishing to speak their secular agendas and humanistic ideas into our identities. Whether emanating from the pressures of the workplace, echoing down the halls of academia, streaming across cyberspace, or droning *ad nauseam* from advertising, they each call out to our insecurities, offering empty promises of happiness and fulfillment. And like the sirens of Greek mythology who lured sailors to shipwreck, so too, such voices can steer us away from understanding our true value, and from living out the abundant life that God intends for us. The aphorism, "no man is an island," is particularly true for the Christian healthcare professional. To maintain an identity in Christ and effectively live out our faith in in the hostile and secular sphere of healthcare, we need the help of fellow Christians. Since God is the divine community of Father, Son, and Holy Spirit in eternal intimate relationship, a central aspect of our image-bearing identity is our relational capacity. Our connectedness to God and to each other mirrors His triune nature and more fully defines our identity. As a result, we are neither inwardly-focussed, stand-alone characters, nor faceless lost-in-the-crowd entities. Being created in the image of the triune God means that we are both distinct persons and inextricably connected to each other. As such, our faith is personal yet not private.

To best protect our identity in Christ, we need to be part of a holy community. We are relational beings and our faith needs holy relationships to thrive. Paul encourages us this way by saying, "Let the message of Christ dwell among you richly as you teach and admonish one another with all wisdom through psalms, hymns, and songs from the Spirit, singing to God with gratitude in your hearts" (Col. 3:16). Holy community can take a variety of forms, including involvement in a church community, Bible study group, Christian outreach, and Christian parachurch organizations. My wife and I have been longtime members of a local Anglican parish, and are actively involved in Bible study groups, as well as numerous church-related ministries, including hospitality, music ministry, and a monthly outreach mission to the homeless in our downtown. We support numerous parachurch organizations, and have been actively involved with the Ezra Institute for Contemporary Christianity (EICC) and the Christian Medical/Dental Association (CMDA). The key issue is that the community be comprised of biblically centered believers who are serious about living out their faith in the day-to-day fray. Nominality won't do. As Dietrich Bonhoeffer said, "Christianity means community through Jesus Christ and in Jesus Christ. No Christian community is more or less than this"[5]

A holy community can provide us needed support in our work and struggles, encouragement to live out our faith and take risk, and accountability to remain biblically faithful with a Christ-centered identity. As Henri Nouwen said, "Christian community is the place where we keep the flame of hope alive among us and take it seriously so that it can grow and become stronger in us."[6]

One form of Christian support that I have found particularly helpful for encouraging my faith walk and protecting my Christ-formed identity is prayer partnership. It's a tremendous gift to be personally prayed for, and a real privilege to pray into another's intimate life circumstances. Built on a relationship of trust, prayer partnership provides an opportunity for vulnerability and more intimate sharing than would be possible or appropriate in a larger gathering. As a result, such relationships can provide more detailed support and timely encouragement than other forms of holy community, and allow room for the Holy Spirit to enter our lives. As Jesus promised, "where two or more are gathered in my name, there am I among them" (Matt. 18:20). Since there's no place to hide, prayer partners can better hold us to account for our activities and help keep us on track and our identities God-focussed. I currently have two prayer partners; one who lives in Edmonton with whom I meet for coffee on mutually convenient evenings, and one who lives across the country with whom I Skype on select Saturday mornings. Both are fellow physicians who have been important role models for me over the years of Christian stewardship and faith integrity. They've also been through the trenches of medical provision, so they know the issues that I face in healthcare, and are familiar with my struggles of work/life balance. Spending time in the Word with them has added depth to my personal faith and given me fresh insight into the priestly calling of medicine.

RESPONDING TO PATIENTS' MISPLACED IDENTITY

A loss of identity is a threat to all who suffer from illness or disability. Our capacity for gainful employment can be lost; our role in the family can be changed; our talents and hobbies that give us joy can be compromised; our physical strength can slip away; and even our appearance can be unrecognizably altered. Illness and disability can make us feel as though we're coming undone and unmask identity crisis.[7]

Being a patient is a difficult business. I never understood just how difficult, until I had my own turn at donning the open-at-the-back, one-size-fits-nobody blue gown, and had to shuffle across the bathroom floor with my intravenous pole in tow. Reminiscent of the scene from *To Kill a Mockingbird* when Atticus says to Scout, "You never really understand a person until you consider things from his point of view [...] until you climb into his skin and walk around in it,"[8] it was the disability that I suffered which provided for me an opportunity to experience some of the challenges that patients endure. Having my external identifiers stripped away by illness shook my world. My infirmity gave me a deep sense of empathy for patients and their struggles with shaken identity, and a certain insight as to how we, as healthcare providers, might reach out to them with care and compassion.

Although the Bible provides the foundation for our understanding of human dignity, and offers a bedrock starting point for medical professionalism and the practice of patient-centered medicine, few people today seem to hold to a personal identity defined by a scriptural narrative. This includes the patients that we are asked to manage. Therefore, it's important that we take the time to identify those who are struggling with broken identities, and be prepared to speak creational truth into their diminished self-understanding. What follows are a series of cases that illustrate how we might winsomely do this with grace and truth.

THE CASE OF A WORK-BASED IDENTITY

I was recently asked to see a long-haul trucker in our Heart Function Clinic whose work-based identity was challenged by heart disease. He was in his early 50s, and had developed ischemic cardiomyopathy related to a recent anteroapical myocardial infarction. His heart damage had caused left ventricular apical remodeling, resulting in mural thrombus formation and necessitating oral anticoagulation. Because of his severely reduced left ventricular function, he required placement of an intracardiac cardioverter defibrillator (ICD), which meant that he would no longer be allowed to use his professional driver's license. Before I saw the patient, one of the nurses warned me that he was quite upset about his inability to drive a truck. This came as no surprise to me, since our ability to work is a common way we find meaning and purpose in our lives.

When I entered the exam room, I saw that he was a burly man with bilateral sleeve tattoos on his crossed arms. After introducing myself and shaking his meaty hand, I sat down and began our conversation by commiserating with him about losing his license. I explained the rationale for the motor vehicle association's stipulation, and then asked him if he owned his own rig, and about his favorite trucking routes. To improve my connection with him, I mentioned that I also have a Class-1 license (which I got as a young adult to improve my summer job prospects, and which I've maintained for just such doctor/patient bonding purposes). To his incredulous look, I pulled out my wallet card for proof. I joked that because I couldn't find a trucking job during the recession of the early '80s, I had to choose medicine instead. This comment made him chuckle and seem to put him at ease. We then discussed his financial concerns and touched upon some of his prospects for alternative employment. As I made arrangements for him to be reviewed by our social services for financial advice and assistance, I mentioned the importance of having things other than work to define us and give our lives meaning. Then, as I took his blood pressure and placed the extra-large cuff around his arm, I commented on his tattoos.

"That's quite some art work you've got on your arms. Did this one over the elbow hurt much when they did it?" I asked.

He nodded and said, "Ya, right over the bone it smarted a little, but the Celtic symbol is important to me. It reminds of my father, so I didn't mind."

Then I asked, "Do you want to see a tattoo that was *really* painful to get?"

33

"What? Don't tell me you've got a tattoo?" he asked in disbelief.

"Yep, and it sure smarted, too," I said, as I pulled up my pant leg to showed him the little Jesus fish I had tattooed above my right ankle.

The contrast between my small tattoo next to his extensive body art was quite comical, and made him laugh out loud and exclaim, "Oh, so you're a Pisces are you?!"

The interchange acted as a further point of connection with the patient. It also gave me the opportunity to share something of my faith. I explained that my tattoo wasn't a sign of the zodiac, but rather a symbol used by the early church to identify fellow Christians. I mentioned that the word *fish* in Greek is *Ichthys*, and represents the acronym, *Jesus Christ, Son of God, Saviour*. And as I straightened my pant leg and returned to my seat, I added, "And it reminds me of my father, too… my Heavenly Father." I then reiterated the importance of understanding our identity beyond our vocation and asked him about his support network.

"Your situation sounds tough," I said. "It's hard to do this life thing on our own. Do you have any family supports, or community involvement… or go to church?" I asked, to which he replied in the negative. So, in the hopes of opening up his supports to some extent, I enrolled him to take part in our cardiac rehabilitation program, and discussed the value of its group teaching sessions and exercise classes.

To help address identity crisis and confusion in our patients, we need to foster a trusting relationship with them and communicate in word and deed that they are significant in our eyes, that we accept them as they are – tattoos and all – and that they are safe and secure with us. We need to counter the lie that their self-worth is contained within their vocation, and look for opportunities to speak words of creational truth into their lives. And to help them broaden their self-understanding, it's important to encourage them to develop their support networks and provide some practical suggestions as to how this might be done.

THE CASE OF DISEASE-BASED IDENTITY REDUCTION

As Christian healthcare professionals, it's important that we strongly dissuade our colleagues from referring to patients in terms of their disease, such as "the hip in room five" or "the left main awaiting bypass." Patients are more than the diseases they may be suffering from and mustn't have their identities reduced in this way. As Sir William Osler once wisely said, "It is much more important to know what sort of a patient has a disease than what sort of a disease has a patient." So, in all of our clinical interactions, we must do our utmost to defend our patient's image-of-God dignity, and look for ways to provide for them a broader sense of their identity, defined beyond the constraints of illness and disability. Although contrary to secular medical education dogma, I have found that extending such discussions into the realm of faith and gently witnessing to patients has been most helpful to rescue their misplaced identities.

One such example was a patient I was asked to see with a pericardial effusion. He was a welder in his late 40s, and long-time smoker. Because of increasing fatigue and dyspnea, he presented to the emergency department, where he was diagnosed with suspected pericardial tamponade. I was called in to confirm the diagnosis and place a pericardiocentesis drainage catheter, as needed. Although he was hemodynamically stable when I examined him, he had clear findings of raised intrapericardial pressures necessitating drainage. As we were getting set up for the procedure, I had the opportunity to talk with the patient, and learned that he had been a former martial arts instructor. To put him at ease while injecting the local anaesthetic, I asked him more about his martial arts training. When he told me that he had attained his *Nidan* second-degree black belt in Karate, I promised to proceed with extra care so as not to provoke him. Then I shared some of my struggles in judo class as a child, and my inability to even proceed past the beginner white belt level.

35

"I'm a lover, not a fighter," I confessed with a smile, and proceeded to drain over a litre of blood-tinged pericardial fluid from his chest.

Some days later, I received a copy of his pathology report. It was bad news. The fluid analysis revealed malignant cells, most likely secondary to adenocarcinoma of the lung. When I saw him on the cardiology ward, he had already been told about his underlying cancer diagnosis and was understandably quite blue. I asked him about the comfort of the pericardial catheter and briefly checked the site to make sure the drain was still operational. Then I sat down next to him and relayed how sorry I was to hear about the diagnosis.

"Guess it's the end of the line for me, Doc," he said weepily. "Never thought it would come done to this, being stuck in a hospital bed, and wasting away as some cancer case."

"I wouldn't give up that easy," I countered. "The road ahead may not be easy, but I'm sure your black belt wasn't handed to you on a platter, either. No doubt you earned it the hard way. Your discipline and fighting spirit will be important to draw from now. Besides, I've been in contact with your oncologist. Sounds like they've got an outpatient treatment regimen planned for you. You should be out of here in no more than a week."

Then I asked him about his support network. He mentioned having a few work buddies and a brother in town, and told me that he had been divorced some years earlier, and that his three children lived with his ex-wife near Toronto.

I shared that I had always wanted daughters, and showed him a photo of my three sons. "Take a look at this bunch of trouble-makers. Do you have any photos of your family?"

He pulled out his phone and showed me a beautiful picture of his children sitting together and smiling.

"That's why all children should be girls," I joked, as I admired his photo. "It would be good for you to have a photo like this on your bedside table," I said to him, and added, "Why don't you send it by email to my secretary? I'll have her print one off for you."

To help broaden his thoughts beyond his disease, I also mentioned that it would be nice to have some visual reminder of his martial arts days, and asked, "What about seeing if your brother can bring in your Karate gi and belt? I'd love to see them, and it would be good to have those reminders of personal discipline in view, particularly as you face the planned investigations and treatments ahead." And then I added with a smile, "And that way none of the other patients or staff will mess with you, either."

When I next visited him, I brought with me a framed copy of the photo of his children and sat it on his dresser. After he thanked me, he pointed to the window curtain where his gi was hung, and said, "Thanks for reminding me that I'm a fighter. I'm gonna beat this cancer."

Then he showed me his blue plastic wristband which had the embossed words, "I make a difference." He told me that his sister-in-law had brought it in for him to wear, along with some others to hand out. As a 'thank-you' for my encouragement, he gave me one. As I rolled up my sleeve to add the band to my collection, he spied my colourful gospel bracelet and asked about its meaning.

I replied, "That's my I.D. bracelet of sorts. It reminds me of who I am and what I'm about." I briefly described what each bead represented, and I asked him if he had ever had any church involvement. He said that he hadn't, but that now was perhaps a good time to start. Then, with his permission, I involved our hospital Chaplain to visit him.

To some extent, all patients are at risk for having their identity reduced by their disease. Facing your own mortality can certainly place in jeopardy your sense of security, acceptance and significance. Even just the prospect of having an ailment can rattle your identity. Some patients

37

develop a disability-based identity, where their symptoms or illness are given a life of their own. In these cases, the diagnosis label sometimes functions to justify an illness, providing the patient a certain rationale for their disabilities. By contrast, without a firm diagnosis, a patient may be left with no real way of making sense of their suffering or communicating their distress to others. While there may be some relief in having a medical pronouncement – like getting a note from home excusing you from having to participate in school gym class – it's a soul-robbing experience to have one's identity reduced to that of a disease state.

THE CASE OF DISABILITY IDENTITY

I had a patient who suffered from a disability identity even though she didn't really have a significant disability. She was a widow in her mid-70s with well-controlled hypertension and a family history of heart disease involving her two brothers of similar vintage. She was an anxious patient who exemplified the *worried well* of our privileged population. I was asked to see her for symptoms of recurrent palpitations, which I felt where related to harmless atrial ectopy. But despite my attempts at reassurance, her symptoms continued, and I was asked to see her again. This time, in addition to her complaints of "having a frog in my chest," she had a two-page list of questions and concerns, largely generated, I suspected, from her online reading. So, after reassuring her that her most recent Holter monitor was also benign, I took her queries in hand, and went through them, one by one, writing my responses in the margin next to each question.

Once she seemed satisfied that she wasn't going to drop dead any time soon, I asked her about her interests and activities (outside of reading Dr. Google, that is). She mentioned that she did some daily walking, and attended a local Roman Catholic parish. I asked her more about her activity level, and to open up her support network, I encouraged her to get involved in group walking. I suggested that she look into the programs offered through the local community recreation centre and even her parish. Then I talked with her about her church supports. After mentioning the importance of church community in my own life and some of my involvements, I encouraged her to get further involved, and suggested she take part in a Bible study and join one of the hospitality groups. As our time together was drawing to a close, I asked if I could pray for her. She seemed delighted with the idea, and so I prayed for her general health and for her understanding that she was a child of God, created in His image, and asked God to calm her anxieties and settle her worries. Then, I wrote out two Scripture references on a prescription pad and said with a smile, "Here's a Scripture script that might be good to follow as directed."

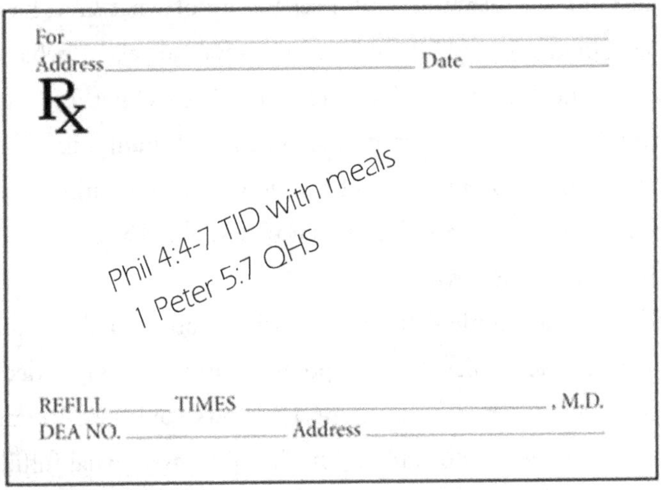

Figure 1. Scripture Script

ADDRESSING SEXUALITY-BASED IDENTITY

Sexual lifestyles and behaviour that contradict the biblical creation narrative are also examples of identity crisis and confusion. The Genesis account provides the primary model for sexuality by which all sexual expressions are understood. Scripture clearly profiles the monogamous life-long marriage relationship of a man and woman as the model for God's character in the expression of intimacy and covenantal love. From a creational standpoint, we understand our gender and sexuality in terms of the Imago Dei revelation, encompassed in the doctrine of the Trinity. Analogous to the distinct Persons of the Godhead all being One God, there is a male and female sacred distinction, where each are separate persons, but "become one flesh" (Gen. 2:24). In this way, the male and female genders are complementary to one another, yet retain separate functions. However, in sexual relationships outside of the biblical model, this all breaks down. Rather than a male and female sacred distinction, there is by contrast, a collapse of gender distinction and a celebration, instead, of a diversity of genders; and in so doing, a joining of what God has separated and a separating of what God has joined. The destigmatization of all forms of non-marital sexual behaviour has produced a no-fault view of sex, reducing it to something casual not covenantal, recreational not procreational, self-gratifying rather than self-giving, and a commodity to be bought and sold, rather than priceless intimacy to be protected. In this way, sexuality has become idolized, and given a life of its own.

While we are undeniably sexual beings, our sexuality should not be our central identifier. Contemporary cultural messages decree that all sexual attractions may represent a person's core identity, and if so, should be celebrated and acted upon. In this sense, sexual fulfillment is considered the end goal of all enterprise. Of course, this distorted linking of sexual behaviour as ultimate fulfillment is doomed to disappointment. No sex experience can meet such dizzyingly high expectations.

By opposing God's design for sexuality, our culture has set into motion an unparalleled identity crisis, and at the same time opened up a giant gospel opportunity for the Christian community to witness God's love to broken people.

My first real exposure to the LGBT community began at the height of the AIDS epidemic in Canada in the mid-1980s. I was a medical student at St. Paul's hospital in downtown Vancouver, and did my clerkship before the introduction of anti-retroviral therapy, when acquiring HIV was akin to being given a death sentence. As a student intern, I directly followed 8 to 10 patients, the majority of whom were gay men about my age, dying of AIDS. It was heart-wrenching to watch their opportunistic infections and cancers progress and, despite our best efforts, consume them. During this training time, while I tried to memorize my differential diagnoses and develop my physical exam techniques, I witnessed the devastation of this pitiless disease on the human condition. William Osler once said, "Know syphilis, and know medicine," but for me it was, *know AIDS, and know the limitations of medicine.* It was a brutal boot camp for learning medicine, to be sure, but the experience gave me on-the-job training in humility and compassion as I worked to respond to the suffering of my patients. As a student, I had a certain luxury of time, and I spent mine not just chasing down lab results and writing up histories, but also at my patients' bedsides with their families, their lovers, and their extensive friend groups. I learned something of the struggles that the gay community faced, their frustrations and brokenness, and their need for acceptance and understanding. So, while I don't pretend to be an expert in the field of LGBT health, I have had formative experiences that have opened my heart to those who label themselves in this way, and have since felt drawn to reach out to them with care and compassion.

Patients who identify as LGBT are at a substantially higher risk for poor health outcomes as compared to the general population. Related to the stigmatization and discrimination that these patients have been subject to in our society, they have been historically less visible and less likely to seek medical attention. While there has since been a growing level of visibility and acceptance for sexual minorities within our society in recent times, many of those within this people group remain underserviced medically. Although significant medical advances have occurred in the past number of decades with, for example, the institution of highly active antiretroviral therapy (HAART) to suppress HIV replication and bring a certain control to the devastation of AIDS infection, significant health issues remain for members of the non-heterosexual community. Not only do they suffer from higher rates of depression, substance abuse, eating disorders, homelessness, and involvement in prostitution; members of this diverse group are more likely to experience sexual abuse, intimate violence, post-traumatic stress disorder, and have a startling 20 times increase in suicide rates.[9] The reluctance to come under medical scrutiny, coupled with their higher prevalence of disease, has resulted in significant health disparities for LGBT patients.

Understanding the scope of health challenges faced by individuals in this people group is an important step in providing them with the care that they deserve. For example, it's important to be aware that gay men and transgender patients, in general, are at a higher risk of sexually transmitted infections, including HIV. Lesbian women tend to more likely struggle with weight gain, and are less likely to have regular cancer screenings. LGBT youth also have particular risks in that they are more likely to experience significant mental health problems, engage in risky behaviors, become the victims of violence, and have a substantially higher risk of suicide, including completed suicide. As well, elderly LGBT patients are at risk for poor social support due to social isolation and generational stigmatization.[10]

Nurturing a trusting healthcare practitioner-patient relationship with our LGBT patients can allow us to not only address the health disparities of this community and reduce health risks, but also speak gentle truth into their confused identity. A Christian response to the LGBT culture is rife with challenges, both on the political front, as we attempt to winsomely defend biblical truth in the public sphere, and on the home front, as we walk alongside and attempt to provide care for those struggling sexually in our personal circle. However, in terms of our professional role towards patients who identify with the LGBT culture, our response is relatively straightforward: we need to welcome these people into our practices with open arms. It's not that we are to celebrate the expression of their sexuality, nor affirm their misdirected identity, but neither is our role to criticize their choices or employ some form of conversion therapy in the hopes of changing them. While there may be certain merits to counseling or spiritual interventions for addressing a patient's gender dysphoria, this isn't our task. Pastors and psychotherapists trained in such matters are better equipped and positioned to do so. Rather, our role is to warmly engage those within the LGBT community with care and concern. To do so, we need to foster a welcoming and sensitive medical atmosphere for them. In terms of *safe spaces*, our clinical environment most certainly should be one. Asking about any special needs or concerns, such as a desire for a chaperone, and providing single-occupant gender-neutral washroom access can go a long way in making patients from this group feel at ease and secure. Detailed resources are available to assist practitioners in the development of a sensitive clinical environment that will better attract and not dissuade LGBT patients, including examples of LGBT-inclusive medical history forms, and culturally-sensitive LGBT patient registration forms, which have inclusive questionnaire options such as separate questions for birth sex and gender.[11]

An easy starting point to establish patient rapport is to learn and use their preferred name. It seems like a simple thing, but means a great deal to patients who are conflicted in this way. Patients who struggle with gender and are experimenting with names are in a very vulnerable position, and desperately want to fit into the gender they've chosen. We can help to diffuse this anxiety by addressing them with their preferred name. I also make use of their preferred name in my correspondence letters with physicians. This allows me to avoid the confusion of pronouns. For example, in a letter regarding a male to female transgendered patient, I would write: "I had the pleasure of reviewing this 47 year-old male-to-female transitioning patient today, who goes by the preferred name of 'Nancy'..." And then for clarity's sake would use the name, "Nancy," or the term, "the patient," instead of pronouns, allowing me to communicate my concerns without compromising biological realities. This is important, since there are significant gender differences that impact our clinical thinking and patient management. In the case of *Nancy*, we can't forget that there's a prostate gland that will require assessment at some point. Or if we consider a female-to-male transitioned patient, we can't forget about cervical cancer screening. As much as men and women share physiology, there are critical differences that we need to be consciously aware of in order to best manage our patients. So, during my interactions with the patient, I go with whatever preferred name they wish, but in my medical communications, written and verbal, I maintain clarity and keep to standard biological nomenclature.

As Christian healthcare professionals, we need to be seen as people who are acutely sympathetic to the deep-seated needs of those who struggle with sexual confusion. After all, it's not *us and them*. Non-heterosexuals are not the enemy. Sexual brokenness is ubiquitous and comes from our sinful nature brought on by the fall and magnified by the sexualized culture in which we're immersed. Consider for a moment the immensity of sexual sin within the heterosexual community, including premarital sex, serial monogamy, masturbation, adultery, and pornography addiction. None of us are *straight*, in a certain sense, but "all like sheep have gone astray" (Is. 53:6). We are all in desperate need of the redemptive work of Christ and sanctifying work of the Holy Spirit, and this is why Christ died. So, next to my gospel bracelet, I wear a rainbow-coloured cloth band with the inscribed letters *WWJD*, which serves as a reminder of my heart for the LGBT community. It also functions as a bit of a conversation starter. If the opportunity arises, the bracelet allows me to share something of my faith, and my concern for the health disparities of this community. The rainbow is our symbol, after all, and is a reminder of God's great promises for all people who come to Him.

CONCLUDING REMARKS

As the preceding cases and concerns illustrate, how we think about ourselves and our identity is intimately tied to our worldview, and can have a direct impact on our health. Our sense of significance, security and acceptance get played out in how we respond to life's challenges – disease and disability included. The origins issue, then, is not merely some abstract philosophy for academics to ponder and debate; it's our very identity that's on the line. It's important to realize that our identity is a creational issue – it's either something that we recognize as created by God, or something understood to be in the realm of our own invention. Whichever origins narrative we accept will end up forming the basis of our self-knowledge, and have a direct bearing on how we try to meet our core needs. The origins narrative influences not only who we understand God to be, but who we understand ourselves to be, which gets played out in the ways we try to find personal significance, acceptance, and security. Since secular thinking pervades the practice of Canadian healthcare, it can be particularly challenging, as a Christian healthcare professional, to maintain a biblically based identity. The concern is this: if we loosen our hold on the creational narrative of Scripture, we risk loosening our hold on our life-giving core identity and succumbing to identity crisis. To keep our biblical faith central in our practice, it's important to intentionally protect our identity in Christ. Immersing ourselves in Scripture and being involved in holy community are important means of guarding ourselves from accepting a lesser understanding of who we are. Bolstered in this way, we are also in a better position to recognize identity crisis and confusion in our patients and look for ways of speaking creational truth into their lives.

SUMMARY POINTS – GOOD CREATION

1. Our identity is a creational issue

2. An identity in Christ requires protection from secular culture's promotion of a self-made identity

3. Being immersed in the Word of God and having an accountability prayer partner are basic means of protecting our identity in Christ

4. We need to address patients' need for security, acceptance, and significance

5. Patients are at risk for disability identity crisis

6. Scripture scripts can remind patients of their true identity

7. Gender and sexuality are best understood in terms of the Imago Dei revelation and the doctrine of the Trinity

8. The LGBT community is a high-risk population with a medical care gap

9. We need to make every effort to foster a welcoming and sensitive medical atmosphere for our LGBT patients

QUESTIONS FOR REFLECTION AND DISCUSSION

1.   How does the biblical creation narrative assist you in understanding your identity?

2.   By what means do you find security in your life? How do you find acceptance in your life and what provides you with a sense of significance?

3.   Have you struggled with a work-based identity or some other identity than Christ?

4.   What steps have you found useful and taken to protect your identity in Christ?

5.   What is your routine for reading the Bible? Are you involved in Bible study?

6.   Why is it important to have a community of faith? Has it been difficult for you to establish a holy community of support?

7.   Do you have a prayer partner? Do you find this provides accountability in your faith life?

8.   Have you had patients who struggled with work-based identity or a disease-based identity? How could you speak words of truth into their lives to help counter this?

9.   What kind of considerations for LGBT patients have you found useful in your practice? What might you need to do to remove the obstacles?

10. What challenges has the LGBT community had for your practice? Do you anticipate any?

11. Are there ways you have strayed from the biblical sexual ethic? Considering the forgiveness that we have received, how shall we then respond to those in the LGBT community?

12. As we consider the tension between biblical truth and compassionate care, have you been too far on one side of the spectrum or the other? Overly condemning? Overly affirming? Consider steps you could take to better maintain the needed balance.

Chapter Notes

1. "Whales are people too: Are we ready to see them as equals?" *Reader's Digest.* July 2012.

2. https://lifechrome.com/tim-keller-quotes

3. Anderson, Neil T. *Living Free in Christ.* Regal Books, 1993.

4. Poortvliet, R. *He was one of us.* Baker Books, 1994.

5. Bonhoeffer, D. *Life Together: The Classic Exploration of Christian Community.* Harper and Row, 1945.

6. Jantz, G. *Soul Care: Prayers, Scriptures, and Spiritual Practices for When You Need Hope the Most.* Tyndale Momentum, 2019.

7. Erikson, E.H. *Identity and the Life Cycle.* New York: International Universities Press, 1959.

8. Lee, Harper. *To Kill a Mockingbird.* Warner Books, 1982.

9. Dhejne, C, et.al. "Long-Term Follow-Up of Transsexual Persons Undergoing Sex Reassignment Surgery: Cohort Study in Sweden." *PLoS ONE,* 2011; 6(2). Affiliation: Department of Clinical Neuroscience, Division of Psychiatry, Karolinska Institutet, Stockholm, Sweden.

10. "Sexuality and Gender: Findings from the Biological, Psychological, and Social Sciences." *The New Atlantis* (Special Report) – Lawrence Mayer and Paul McHugh. August 2016 (http://www.thenewatlantis.com/publications/number-50-fall-2016).

11. *Fenway Guide to Lesbian, Gay, Bisexual & Transgender Health,* 2nd Edition.

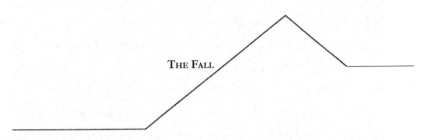

THE FALL

CHAPTER 2

DISTRESS AND DESPAIR

"Why is light given to those in misery, and life to the bitter of soul, to those who long for death that does not come, who search for it more than for hidden treasure, who are filled with gladness and rejoice when they reach the grave?"

Job 3:20-2

THE LOSS OF MEANING IN SUFFERING

The fall is the second feature of the gospel contour, and is placed on the conflict or rising action line along the biblical narrative. The conflict, of course, is man's rejection of God's command – the solitary prohibition symbolizing Yahweh's supreme authority – as an intentional attempt

53

to "be like God, knowing good and evil" (Gen. 3:4). And the rising action that follows is the direct result of this forfeited fellowship with God, and separation from the abundant life He offers. Every one of us is affected by this fallen human condition. As Aleksandr Solzhenitsyn, Russian novelist, moralist, and gulag survivor wisely observed, "The battle line between good and evil runs through the heart of every man."[1] This essential element of the gospel message provides the foundation for why things are awry and points to our need for a Saviour. Rather than an isolated incident, this portion of the gospel narrative represents a comprehensive effect, involving all aspects of creation, and every sphere of our culture, including the health of our bodies and the practice of medicine. As anyone working in healthcare would agree, despite our diagnostic acumen, technical wizardry, and scientific advances, we remain perpetually stymied by disease, death, and decay. Likewise, one look around ourselves, as well as any honest look in the mirror, clearly shows that brokenness has affected us all – patients and practitioners alike – and that we're all in need of wholeness and healing.

Our secularized culture flatly rejects this gospel narrative and views the biblical fall as an antiquated myth. In exchange, our society has accepted *chance* as an explanation for why what goes down goes down. Numerous Christians also minimize the doctrine of the fall, reducing it to little more than an ancient poem or Sunday school story. Insulted by the suggestion that they should take the account literally, many fail to take it seriously. There is mystery here, to be sure. But to write off the first chapters of Genesis on the basis of poetic language and narrative format creates more problems than mere interpretative strain. If we neglect the fall, we forfeit the basis for the sinful condition of humankind. This sets us up to believe the lie that everyone is essentially *good*, and figure that "man is born to trouble as surely as sparks fly upwards" (Job 5:7) simply because of chance operating in their lives.

54

The central limitation of choosing chance as an explanation for reality is simply that it can't explain reality – it lacks causative agency. Although chance has been given a life of its own in our secular narrative, it remains merely an immaterial notion. As such, chance has no operative capacity and can do nothing to directly affect the material world. While the play of chance is a useful concept for understanding the probability of events, chance, as an entity, is a total myth. While there may be a fifty-fifty *chance* that a coin flipped into the air will land heads-up, *chance* can't cause the coin to land this way. There are a certain number of variables that are at play to contribute to the toss outcome, including the coin's starting position, the force exerted by the thumb producing the flipping action, the firmness of the landing surface, and so on. However, chance, as a non-force, does nothing more than imply the relative statistical likelihood of a particular result. Despite this, however, the acceptance of chance is well-entrenched in our society and likely explains the widespread adoption of fatalism and superstitious behaviours in our culture. This may be because, in a pure chance environment, superstitious rituals create the illusion of control and certainty. From blowing on the dice to achieve a winning roll, or saying "good luck" or "touch wood" to ensure a good outcome, such behaviours seem to give people a sense that they've done one more thing to stack the odds in their favor. As irrational as avoiding walking under ladders or crossing paths with a black cat to avoid future catastrophe, the embrace of a false certainty functions for many as a surrogate for real certainty.

This is the case in medical culture as well. For example, we routinely avoid saying things like, "Sure is *quiet* in the Emerg," or "*slow* in the clinic day" for fear of putting a *jinx* on the patient flow. As well, many in healthcare hold firmly to the notion that the full moon "brings out the neurotics and worst trauma cases," and medical trainees often talk about having "good call Karma" if they don't get paged much overnight. And, because of its connotation with *bad luck*, the number 13 has intentionally been omitted from designating hospital elevator numbering, ward rooms or operating theatres. Who would want to undergo the knife in operating room number thirteen, after all? ... Especially if it were a Friday with forecast for a full moon!

Although when pressed, most would deny actually believing in such irrational superstitions, these types of ritualistic behaviours betray a deep-seated fear of the future and a fatalistic *modus operandi* for the present. This shouldn't surprise us. If the doctrine of the fall is loosely held, so too is the doctrine of salvation, and any real hope for a remedy to the troubles of this world, including our own struggles and suffering. As such, those who hold to a chance view of the world are left to coddle superstitious rituals and horror-scope predictions, and are understandably prone to suffer from anxiety and fear about future possibilities. Without a firm belief in God's promises and providence, and the genuine conviction that he is present at all times – particularly during times of trial and troubles – people are more liable to experience distress and despair when coming onto hard times and, so-called, "bad luck."

DEATH WISH OF DESPAIR

This was certainly my problem before my stroke. I had a rather trivialized view of the fall, and as a result, I had an incomplete appreciation for the divine remedy available for me. I considered that the events of my day largely unfolded by happenstance, rather than by God's providence. And if events remarkably concurred, I would put it down to mere coincidence, and let God-incidences go unnoticed. When a problem would arise, like work pressure, financial difficulty, or a strained relationship, I would approach it in the same fashion as any of my secular colleagues, and never think of taking it to the Lord in prayer. I didn't seem to be any worse for wear from my worldly thinking until illness struck. Then, due to my lack of appreciation for the fall and its intimate connection with personal salvation, I found myself unprepared to deal with my personal suffering.

Although I made a miraculous recovery after the stroke, I continued to struggle with repetitive bouts of intense fatigue, which sapped my get-up-and-go like a hot humid day. I'd frequently have to stop what I was doing for lack of energy and just lie down. It reminded me of the time when I hit the 20-mile wall at the Boston Marathon. And similar to that steep portion of Heartbreak Hill, the fatigue posed a seemingly insurmountable obstacle to my rehabilitation efforts. Lying down and resting did little to relieve the pain of it, and sometimes only seemed to make it worse for lack of distraction. During those episodes, I struggled to find any meaning in my suffering, and as time wore on, I became increasingly demoralized and depressed.

One evening, after I'd forced myself off the couch for a change of scene, I dressed for a walk through the neighborhood in the hopes of energizing myself. It was early winter with a forecast for snow, so I donned my parka and boots. It felt good to get out, stretch my legs, and breathe in the crisp night air. So, to extend my walk, I made my way down the hill from our house to a quiet field next to a farm. It was so peaceful and quiet, I decided to lie down on my back in the snow. Staring up at the night sky, there was no moon to comfort nor stars to orientate, just the deep black abyss. I felt a heavy emptiness overcome me. Then, in response to a growing frustration that had been brewing since the stroke, I said aloud,

"Take me now, Father... I've got nothing more I can do... I'm so tired, I just feel done... Just take me now, please. I want to die!"

I felt like George Bailey from *A Wonderful Life*, at the end of my rope, and sick and tired of being of being sick and tired. My energy level was at a record low and my motivation to carry on had disappeared. I wasn't sure if I'd be able to return to any meaningful work. Everything just seemed so bleak and meaningless. I just wanted it all to end. So, I continued to lay there in the field with eyes closed, and repeated my death wish a few more times, half hoping, I guess, to be taken up in a whirlwind like Elijah or something. I'm not sure how much time went by. I must've dozed off a bit, because when I finally opened my eyes, I was wearing a thin layer of freshly-fallen snow. The wind had picked up and the snow was gusting around me. So, I got up, brushed off the snow and muttered, "Die another day," as I plodded uphill home.

Although I didn't have suicidal ideation and any need for the suicide prevention helpline, the dark despair that had gripped me during that time of struggle could've certainly led down that desperate path. The vacuum of anguish can be overwhelming to experience, and not surprisingly, can cause its sufferers to question the value of their lives and long for death. Suicide prevalence on the planet is staggering. With nearly one million deaths each year, suicide takes a tragic toll on global public health. The statistics in our society are no less shocking, particularly amongst our young-adult population. Right on the heels of motor vehicle accidents, suicide is the leading cause of death for those aged 15 to 34 years of age, and a grim reminder as to the existential suffering that many in this demographic painfully experience.[2] Despite the steady mortality decline achieved for all the other major causes of death in North America like heart disease and cancer, suicide rates continue to climb annually. Although these statistics are disturbing enough, the rates are probably an underestimate. Frequently suicides go unreported, and many are disguised as "accidental deaths."

Adding to the heartbreak of suicide is that the decision is often impulsive. It's been well-documented that those who survive their attempt at self-extinction consistently express profound suicidal regret – even in the process of the act. In the documentary film, "Suicide: the Ripple Effect," Kevin Hines – a survivor of a Golden Gate Bridge suicide jump – said that the moment his fingers left the rail, "I realized I made the greatest mistake of my life." And his case is not an isolated one. The majority of suicidal crises are self-limiting, evidenced by the fact that more than 90% of people who survive a suicide attempt don't try again.[3] As well, the fallout far exceeds the tally of those who commit this ultimate self-harm. For every victim of suicide, there are dozens of devastated family members, friends, colleagues, roommates and acquaintances left behind. As detailed in his book, *Grieving Suicide*, Albert Hsu discusses the psychological trauma experienced by the surviving family members, and places it on par with trauma sustained from surviving a terrorist attack, and as scarring as a soldier's experience in combat.[4]

Suicide occurs tragically enough in the medical community, as well. Although seldom discussed in medical circles, doctors have a suicide rate that is estimated to be three times higher than that of the general population. Long hours, overwhelming workload, and lack of support are among the factors pushing physicians past burnout to bursting. An estimated 400 physicians commit suicide in the U.S. each year.[5] Two of my classmates killed themselves while established in their professional lives, as did a prominent cardiologist I trained under, as well as two other well-recognized heart specialists who I knew. Reminiscent of the narrative poem, *Richard Cory* – who "was rich – yes, richer than a king – and admirably schooled in every grace… So on we worked, and waited for the light, and went without the meat, and cursed the bread; and Richard Cory, one calm summer night, went home and put a bullet through his head"[6] – their worldly successes and affluence did nothing to protect them from life's bitter despair.

THE NEED FOR A THEOLOGY OF SUFFERING

Healthcare provision can be fraught with stressors: the time pressures are constant; the problems complex; patients' needs can seem never-ending; our best efforts can go unnoticed, and patient outcomes can be unsatisfying, sometimes even tragic. If given the opportunity, all-consuming distress and despair can easily get the best of us. So, it's important to take care. As the apostle Peter warns, we need to "Be alert and of sober mind. Your enemy the devil prowls around like a roaring lion looking for someone to devour" (1 Pt. 5:8). If we are to keep our faith in the forefront of our medical practice, then intentional measures are required to protect ourselves from the risk of either becoming calloused of heart or burned out in soul. It's important to have a well-developed theology of suffering that can withstand both the travails of our patients, as well as our own.

Everyone – whether a healthcare professional or layperson, a Christian believer or not – needs to address the problem of pain and suffering to some degree and in some fashion. As Immanuel Kant stated, "evil is a personal challenge to every human being and can be overcome only by faith."[7] For Christian worldview defense, there are detailed and persuasive works on the topic of theodicy which outline how, indeed, God can be all-powerful and all-loving, and yet allow evil and suffering. However, there is little room for such discussions in the realm of clinical medicine. While there is merit to being familiar with theodicy arguments, and to "be prepared to give an answer to everyone who asks you to give the reason for the hope that you have" (1 Pt. 3:15), at the bedside of those grieving, it's not about debating or argument, but listening and care. When dealing with patients and families who are in the throes of anguish, our role is to come alongside them in their suffering. For them, the issue of suffering is not an intellectual exercise to be grappled with, but an experiential ache that needs comforting. The problem with pain is that it hurts. As Christian healthcare professionals, we are called to enter into these dark places with compassionate care and shine the light of Christ.

Our best protection from the spectre of suffering and evil is the cross of Christ. By this, I don't mean holding up a wooden crucifix as portrayed in B-movies to ward off vampires. Rather, in order to best face the distress and despair of medicine, it's important to have a clear understanding as to the significance of the cross in our daily lives. The biblical answer to pain is not one of stoic indifference, denial, or defeat. God has not abandoned us to despair. The problems of evil and suffering are ultimately answered by God's intimate involvement in the human condition at the cross. Martin Luther said, "When you look around and wonder whether God cares, you must always hurry to the cross and you must see Him there."[8]

Jesus knows about suffering in all its manifestations, and is well-acquainted with grief and hardship. Born into poverty, in His lifetime He experienced thirst, hunger, fatigue and temptation. He knew what it felt like to be bullied, dismissed by family, and betrayed by friends. He was ridiculed and taunted, scorned and spat upon, whipped and beaten, and publically humiliated in the raw exposure of execution. He was, indeed, "a man of sorrows, and familiar with suffering. Like one from whom men hide their faces, He was despised and rejected" (Is. 53:3). By freely allowing Himself to be crucified, Jesus hallowed earthly pain and gave us an example of suffering in obedience to the Father's will. As a result of His suffering, we can meet Him in ours. As our mediator, Jesus is the way we get to God, and the way God gets to us. With the crucifixion, God turned the cruelest instrument of execution the world had known, into the symbol of covenantal love, recognized the world over. Just as God made use of His Son's suffering to claim back humanity with salvation, He can also make use of our bodily suffering to display His

61

good works. As Malcolm Muggeridge said, "Everything that has truly enhanced and enlightened my existence has been through affliction."[9] While suffering is not our only portal of entry to God, it's a sure and certain one, and one to remember when we are in the midst of struggle. Because of the cross, we can be confident that our suffering does not go unnoticed nor is senseless, but has eternal meaning and value.

Although I grew up in the church, I didn't spend much time dwelling on Christ's suffering and its significance for my life. As a child, Good Friday was *good* because it was a school holiday, and Easter was less about Christ's passion and more about my own passion for chocolate bunnies and candy egg scavenger hunts. Even as an adult, in my eagerness to celebrate Easter, I would rush through Holy Week to quickly get to the party part. Who wants to perseverate over Friday's grief and sorrow when there's so much Sunday triumph and praise awaiting? But of course, Resurrection Sunday has little meaning without Good Friday. Unless we appreciate the sacrifice and suffering of Jesus, we are less likely to believe that what He accomplished on the cross was real or relevant for us today. Without a deep sense of His passion and its significance, our theology of suffering becomes superficial and little different from that of secular disdain. After all, in our contemporary culture, there is no hallowing of suffering. In our euthanasia-permissive society, pain is not only a four-letter word, it's considered a menace to be eliminated at any cost, even if that cost is the life of the sufferer.

HOLDING TIGHT TO THE CROSS OF CHRIST

In order to remember that God has not abandoned me to my suffering, I have a number of ways of keeping Christ's passion fixed in the forefront of my mind. During the Holy Week of Easter, for example, I celebrate a Christian version of the Seder meal with my family. The traditional meal incorporates various symbols of the Hebrews' slavery in Egypt. The ritual of repeatedly eating pieces of broken flat bread and sipping red wine has given me a deeper appreciation for the significance of Holy Communion and the rich symbolism of Jesus as the Passover Lamb. In addition to this practice, I make a point of watching Mel Gibson's film, *The Passion of the Christ* during the Easter season. Although this brutally violent depiction of Jesus' last hours is not for the faint of heart, I've found it a spiritually-poignant experience. Despite the fact that the movie is a bit like being barked at by a dog for two hours, the annual viewing shellshocks me into deep gratitude, and more fully prepares me for Easter Sunday's triumphant celebrations. Remembering His death this way, I am in a better position to not only celebrate the resurrection of Christ, but to eagerly await His promised return.

To keep Christ's passion in my mind beyond Easter and through the whole year, I make a point of regularly meditating on the Stations of the Cross. There's a local prayer garden where the Stations are portrayed, which is ideal for reflective walks. As well, I've set up my own meandering path in the back woods at our cottage, which demarcates the memorials of Jesus' final hours. I've found this liturgical practice a rich one. Retracing the route of Jesus, from Gethsemane to Golgotha, gives structure to my prayers and meditation, and allows me to consider my experiences of human suffering in their proper context. With the cross in mind, I take my failed resuscitation responses, grief-filled patient encounters, and emotional quiet-room discussions, as well as personal struggles, and give them over to Christ to bear for me, as only He is able to do.

Lastly, to center my day-to-day walk on Christ's passion, I wear a small wooden cross around my neck. Hidden under my shirt and tie, no one need be aware of this ancient symbol but me. From the early morning, when I place it around my neck, to the late evening hours, when I hang it with my shirt and tie set out for the next day, it brings to mind God's unfathomable sacrificial love. Regardless of the stress and strain of my workday, the cross reminds me I'm not alone. As I feel its smooth contour pressing against my chest, I am reassured that Jesus knows about my suffering and wants to meet me there. And I don't always just keep it quietly tucked away. Wearing a cross gives me an easy connect with patients who also wear one. I intentionally comment on theirs, remarking on its beauty and asking where they got it from. Then, quite naturally, I show them my simple cross, and in so doing, open up a faith discussion opportunity.

PRAYER JOURNAL PROTECTION

Keeping a prayer journal is an important spiritual discipline that can foster a maturing of faith and provide a defence from distress and despair. Confiding with God in written word allows us to communicate with Him on a deeper level. It's not that our scribbles tell God anything He doesn't already know, of course; Scripture informs us that God knows our thoughts before a word is on our tongue (Ps. 139:4). However, prayer journaling can give *us* insights into things that we either didn't know, or have forgotten. Sometimes, just the simple process of laying out our thoughts and unpacking our concerns can be therapeutic. It's important that we don't keep things bottled up to bursting. Prayer journaling can function as a useful and healthy outlet for needed expression. But what sets prayer journaling apart from simply keeping a diary, is that this form of written expression is God-directed. As we confide in Him and allow His word to interact with our paragraphs and pages, we invite the Holy Spirit to speak truth into our struggles. Over time, a remarkable thing happens. When we reflect on prior entries, and see how our past troubles have worked out, we can begin to see God's hand in our lives. Such life-giving epiphanies can enable us to better trust Him with our present problems, and place our hopes in him for the future.

I've kept a diary since childhood. At that time, the entries were brief bits of factual information about highlights from my day, along the lines of, "Dear Diary, it rained today, so I played *Snakes-and-Ladders* with Billy at his house." In my teen and young adult years, though, my journaling developed past base expression. I recorded my thoughts and feelings and found that the process, although done sporadically, provided me clarity of thought and an opportunity to gain perspective on my circumstances. As my faith walk matured, my journaling became more of a regular part of my week and took on a prayer-like quality. Complete with confessions, requests, and thanksgiving, the process expanded my morning devotionals from the private expression of piety into the practical engagement of my daily issues. Over the years, I've compiled numerous journal volumes, which take up an increasingly large portion of my office bookshelf.

The immense value of these old prayer journals became evident to me on the evening of my snowy death-wish appeal. After I'd put my parka and boots away, and grabbed a cup of tea to warm myself, I sat in my office to write a journal entry. As I began to do so, my thoughts became interrupted by an impulse to review my older journals. I initially dismissed the urge as some nostalgic whim of little value, and tried to pen my frustrations about my debilitating fatigue. However, as the idea of reviewing the old journals nagged on, I decided to humor myself, and grabbed one off the shelf. Thumbing through its pages, I was struck by how quickly I was transported back in time. Reading the old entries brought back memories as vivid as yesterday. As I did this, I came across numerous challenges and struggles which I had faced in the past, and many of which I'd completely forgotten about. However, reading them with the advantage of hindsight, I was able to recognize how each of those struggles had now resolved. The finding gave me pause. So I took another journal off the shelf, and then another. And each time I did so, I discovered the same phenomenon: my past struggles – which at the time had consumed me – had resolved, oftentimes quite surprisingly, and more wonderfully than I could've wished for. Then *Eureka!* It struck me: God had not abandoned me in my troubles. There on the loose-leaf pages before me was tangible evidence of God's active involvement in my life. Woven through my recorded struggles and strife was a divine thread, linking orchestrated events that were far beyond what I could've asked for or imagined.

Bolstered by this fresh realization, I returned to my current journal entry with renewed vigour and confidence. I wrote down the simple question, "Dear Lord, how should I face my fatigue?" and boldly drew a large circle on the page just below the question, leaving it empty for God's reply. Then, some weeks later, while going through my devotional Scriptures, two verses popped out at me. The first was from the book of Nehemiah, written as consolation for the weeping Israelites, and read, "Do not grieve, for the joy of the Lord is your strength" (Neh. 8:10). The second was from the Song of Moses and Miriam reading, "The Lord is my strength and my song; he has become my salvation. He is my God, and I will praise him, my father's God, and I will exalt him" (Ex. 15:2). I knew immediately that these holy words were the answer to my journal query. It then dawned on me that the enjoyment of the Lord's presence is the only real strength I need – and not even brain fatigue can take that from me – and that my response to fatigue needs to be one of God-directed praise. So, I flipped through my journal again and found my earlier entry, and wrote down the verses in the circle. Now, when I'm hit with bouts of recurring fatigue, I turn to them for encouragement. In this way, rather than grieving over my sapped strength, I reflect on the beauty of God's holiness and revel in my communion with His intimate holy presence.

From that time forward, my journals have taken on a strictly prayerful focus. On its pages, I direct all my penned thoughts and feelings towards God. If I have concerns, I lay them out before Him. This is because it's not just a one-way communication, me-to-God. I also listen for his voice to speak truth into my troubles. I do this by continually posing explicit questions in my journal and requesting His response. Specifically, I write down my query or concern with date and time, and draw a palm-sized circle on the page below the entry in anticipation of His answer. Then, in keeping with the Psalmist who wrote, "In the morning, O Lord, you hear my voice; in the morning I lay my requests before you and wait in expectation" (Ps. 5:3), I also wait in expectation for the Lord's reply. Although some patience is required, I've never been disappointed. Sometimes His reply arrives promptly, even within short minutes; other times it can take weeks or months to get an answer. However long the wait, when the answer comes to mind, I find the corresponding blank circle under my original journal entry, and write it down with a new date and time in the margin. In this way, I can more intentionally track God's intimate involvement in my day-to-day struggles, and prove to myself that God does not abandon me in my troubles, but listens and responds to my concerns.

"How can I be certain that the so-called 'responses' come from God and aren't merely the product of the monkey in my mind?" one might skeptically ask. And while it's possible that there may be an element of wishful thinking taking place here, the responses that I've prayfully received aren't ones that I would've necessarily anticipated, or at times even desired. Furthermore, they have been consistent with the voice of Scripture, which I have come to recognize as the Lord's own. God says, "Call to me and I will answer you, and will tell you great and hidden things that you have not known" (Jer. 33:3). So, while I recognize that this type of evidence is not the same as the empirical proofs we have in the sciences, it is as important. Even though I appreciate the difference between my prayer journal "*aha moments*" and the unbroken uniformity of gravity, for example, I also know that in matters of personal faith, such empirical proof is neither possible nor necessary. As C. S. Lewis clarified, "prayer is request. The essence of request, as distinct from compulsion, is that it may or may not be granted."[10] If the Bible is true, and the Holy Spirit indwells us, then it should be no surprise that God would answer prayer, and no proof beyond this should be necessary.

COUNTERING DISTRESS WITH GOALS OF CARE

As Christian healthcare professionals, we need to be sure and certain that we are not abandoned in our troubles. Patients also need to know this. Feelings of abandonment and helplessness are commonly experienced by patients, and can allow fear to take hold and escalate into distress and despair. We can help counteract this. However, to do so, we need to be prepared to slow down a bit and take some time with our patients. Fears will often dissipate if patients feel that they are being listened to and that their concerns are being taken seriously. During such encounters, we need to provide them with clear medical explanations, and make every effort to involve them in their therapeutic care. This is particularly the case during serious illness presentations and end-of-life management decisions. Discussing goals-of-care with patients is an ideal opportunity to do this. These discussions directly involve patients in their medical plan, and position them as the key player. This can not only moderate their fear, but also diminish distress and despair, and in some instances, even lead to fruitful conversations about life's meaning and purpose and God's promises and providential plan.

The formalized goals-of-care designations we routinely use today are a relatively recent development. During my medical training years, we didn't have such documents to describe and communicate the general aim of patient management. The medical ethos then was very much an approach focussed on *cure*, with very little emphasis placed on the "softer" quality of life *care* issues. At that time, we held to a dichotomy between so-called "active" and "non-active" treatment arms. The former group were the "full code" patients – the ones who would receive curative management efforts, including measures to prolong life with resuscitation and intensive care monitoring, if required. The latter, by contrast, were the "no code" patients, or "DNR" (do not resuscitate) group. They were the patients who had either exhausted all treatment options, and were, as we'd callously say, "sweet-outa-luck," or they had a terminal condition or a poor quality of life, as determined by the attending physician. These patients were categorized by what they *wouldn't receive*, like resuscitative measures, intensive care monitoring or surgical intervention, and not by the symptom control and comfort measures that they *could receive*. At that time, physicians chose one of these two mutually-exclusive management options, and patients and their families were seldom involved in the decision-making.

The binary approach was a straightforward patient management algorithm and relatively easy for us trainees to follow. It was simple: there were either *full-code patients* or *DNR's*. For the former group, you pulled out all the stops and provided immediate, full-resuscitative response, as necessary. For the latter group, by contrast, there was no need for an urgent response should their condition deteriorate. You could just stand back and let nature take its course. However, this over-simplified approach had its problems. Grey-zone cases cropped up now and again, where patients would sometimes fall between the cracks of the two response options. As a cardiology resident, I can painfully recall numerous inappropriate resuscitations I was involved with, where our efforts were futile from the get-go due to the patient's end-stage illness and frailty. I remember just as painfully, numerous examples of patients who might well have benefited from certain intensive interventions, but didn't receive them because of their disabilities or their perceived poor quality of life. I also recall "slow-code" cases, where it was nuanced that the house staff should respond to a patient's cardiac arrest without rushing. We were to go through the motions and not be worried about the poor outcome. This was done largely to fulfill hospital protocol, and obviate the need for the more difficult doctor/patient end-of-life discussion. An even greater concern with this binary approach was how it influenced the way we thought about patients and their value. We adopted either a "full code, full care" stance for patient management, or a "no code, no care" one. This attitude negatively affected not only our nighttime call responses to patients, but also our daytime patient interactions.

With these lingering memories, I celebrated the establishment of our present-day goals-of-care designations. Having a patient-centered treatment overview clearly specified on every hospital chart represents an important step forward in patient care. The continuum of care choices offers a clear advance over the former binary options. The contemporary designations allow for better alignment of patient wishes with the medical management plan, and place increased emphasis on symptom management and compassionate care. Additionally, these patient-centered goals-of-care are in closer concordance with a Christian view of medical practice. We believe that patients are created in the image of God and have inherent value. It directly follows, then, that all patients should be treated with dignity and be involved in a holistic and compassionate healthcare plan. Although the goals-of-care designations may have been driven by medical humanism, it is only the theological doctrine of *Imago Dei* that can supply the needed foundation to make sense of them.

Unfortunately, despite the mandated use of goals-of-care, inadequate communication still persists between healthcare professionals and patients. Issues of concern remain, such as forms not being completed in a timely fashion, or completed incorrectly. As well, goals-of-care discussions are often done on the fly, when physicians are under time pressure. When rushed, these discussions can get reduced to little more than a base transactional contact. And even worse, sometimes these discussions take on an adversarial overtone, particularly if goal disagreements arise between provider and patient. This is shameful and largely avoidable. Defining goals-of-care with patients can be challenging, to be sure, but they represent fertile soil for holistic patient care. These discussions can not only help us foster a compassionate care plan, the process can also provide the opportunity for spiritual discussions to take place. To illustrate this, the following are a series of cases which deal with some of these challenges and highlight some opportunities.

THE CASE BETWEEN THE ROCK AND RESUSCITATION

I was recently involved in a case that illustrates the importance of timely and thorough goals-of-care discussions. My patient was a former boiler-maker in his mid-70s who had end-stage heart disease. Originally from Newfoundland, he was transferred down to our hospital from Fort McMurray where he had been previously working. He had severe aortic valve stenosis complicated by congestive heart failure and was sent to us for interventional consideration. Unfortunately, on account of his severe emphysema, superimposed on his diabetes, peripheral vascular disease, and renal failure, he was not a candidate for either surgical or percutaneous valve intervention. This left only palliative medical management for his valve disease. Reviewing his case, I noticed that there was a full-resuscitative "R1"goals-of-care designation on his hospital chart. Considering his inoperable end-stage condition, I wondered if this was appropriate, and made a mental note to discuss his goals of care with him at some point.

When I walked into his room, he was sitting by the window. Seeing me, he started to get up to walk to his bed. However, I waved him down and said, "Stay where you're to, 'til I comes where yours at." He chuckled as I pulled up a chair next to him. I introduced myself as a fellow Maritimer, telling him that I was a Bluenoser born in Halifax. Then, although I wanted to eventually address his goals-of-care, I opened our discussion with some general rapport-building questions. You can't rush this. Rather than bluntly asking, "are you sure you want everything?" like someone might ask at a hamburger stand, I inquired about his general activities and family life. I learned that he had lived a pretty hard life with heavy drinking and smoking, both of which he'd "come clean of," and that he had a brother and sister "back on the Rock," whom he missed a great deal. I then asked him about his understanding of his heart disease, and in particular, what he had been told by his treating physicians. In response, he said that he'd heard he had a heart murmur, and that he suspected it was bad, but he had no clear idea just how serious. So, I took some time to review his diagnosis with the aid of a diagram, which I drew for him. I discussed with him frankly about the gravity of his condition and the limited options available. To give him some time to process the hard news, I decided to defer addressing his goals-of-care designation until a later time. I finished by encouraging him to inform his family in Newfoundland about his condition, and asked him to write down any questions that might arise, so that I could address them during my next patient rounding.

When I saw him on the following day, he was chatting on Facetime with his sister from the Maritimes. He pointed his phone screen toward me, and introduced me as "the guy who explained *awl dose tings* with the picture." Seeing an opportunity for family involvement, I asked if it would be okay to discuss his medical issues with his sister, to which he nodded in the affirmative. So, I asked him about his goals-of-care, wording it this way: "Knowing about your illness and the limitations of what we can do to halt its progression, what's most important to you? What are you hoping we can do for you?"

His answer was plain enough, "I just wanna go home, Doc… to be with my family. It's all I want, and there's nothing more that can be done for me, here, anyhow. No offense, but I'm tired of being cooped up in a hospital room like this."

I reviewed the goals-of-care document with the patient and his sister, and asked them if it would be helpful for me to offer a recommendation. With his agreement, I made the suggestion that his goals-of-care designation be changed from *resuscitative* to *medical* and that our efforts be focussed on symptom management. They both seemed very pleased with that plan, and started talking about a family reunion. Recognizing that he was in no present condition to fly across the country, I asked him if he wanted to be transferred back to Fort McMurray until he was well enough to travel. He responded that he'd prefer to be back up north. At that point, I asked about his support network there. "Do you have friends there… people who can give you a hand… or connections in the community…? Do you attend church?"

"I have a number of friends in the Fort," he chuckled, "but I've never darkened the door of a church… it would probably collapse if I did." Then, directing his comment to his phone screen, he added, "But my sister here goes to church, and she's a real prayer warrior, aren't you, Sis?"

I concluded our time together by promising to make arrangements for the transfer of his care, and asked the sister if she'd like to pray now. She was eager to oblige, and prayed over us across cyberspace.

It's important to have a clear understanding of our patients' care goals, so we can best align the care provided with their wishes. This is particularly the case in the context of a serious illness among hospitalized patients.[11] Even though these conversations can be difficult, it's essential that we, as Christian healthcare professionals, take this role seriously and make it a priority of doing well. Although goals-of-care decisions are most often completed during hospital admission, they shouldn't be limited to this timing. If undertaken in the outpatient setting, they can be developed over a longer period, and carefully considered in consultation with family members and the primary care physician. End-of-life and goals-of-care discussions initiated by healthcare professionals can also invite a broader discussion within the patient's family about these issues, opening up the topic for them, where it may have been difficult or ignored before.

Discussions about goals of care shouldn't be limited to end-of-life management preferences, focusing only on death and dying, but broadened further to address priorities for living. There's opportunity here to address important issues, and we can use these discussions as a chance to go deeper with our patients and discuss matters of faith. For example, we can follow the standard goals-of-care question, "Do you have personal beliefs that influence your health care wishes?" with further questions that respectfully explore a patient's spirituality, such as, "Do you have a faith community" or "What are your thoughts about life after death?" In this way, the mandated care form moves us closer to Christ's mandate to bear gospel witness. To do this well, we need to have one ear listening to the nudging of the Holy Spirit. It's a bit like having two parallel conversations going simultaneously; one with the patient, as we listen to their concerns, and one with the Holy Spirit, as we lean on His counsel on how to best respond to them. This constant openness to God positions us to be His hands and feet more effectively and to address patients' deeper needs in addition to the surface issues. In this way, discussing goals of care can allow us to provide the very best of care.

The Case of Goals of Care & the Cross

To illustrate an out-patient goals-of-care discussion, I had a case of a patient in her early 60s whom I was asked to see in clinic regarding palpitations. She had a history of hypertension and dyslipidemia, which both seemed to be well-managed on her present medications. Her investigations showed that her heart function was normal and her 24-hour Holter monitor was benign. So, given those reassuring results, I wasn't too concerned about any serious cardiac etiology for her symptoms. As I asked her my routine questions about caffeine consumption, sleep quality, and psychological stressors, she said, "Yes, there's been stress.... overwhelming stress, in fact" and then told me that her eldest daughter had recently committed suicide by hanging. I froze. Her matter-of-fact mention of the tragedy took me completely off guard. Lost for words, I put my pen down and quietly listened to her story. She told me that her daughter had been a varsity athlete and a good student, but had suffered from bouts of depression over the years. Various medications had been tried, and she seemed to be coping reasonably well. Her death came as a shock to everyone. She said that her daughter's body had been discovered by a roommate, who had immediately called the ambulance. Because the attendants were able to resuscitate her daughter, there was some initial hope she might survive. However, after a grueling three days in the intensive care unit on life-support, the family was informed that their beloved was brain dead. With that news, they unanimously agreed to disconnect her from life-support, and allow nature to take its course.

At that point in her story, my patient sobbed into her handkerchief. I had to wipe my own eyes, as well. After a pause, I responded by saying that "I can't imagine what it's been like for you and your family to go through all of this...I'm really very sorry." Then, after a further pause, I tried to reassure her about her own health. I said that I didn't think her palpitations were related to anything wrong with her heart, and that her symptoms were part of a grief response. To wrap things up, I asked her if she had any questions for me. She answered by saying that watching her daughter on the ventilator was traumatizing, and that she would never want to put her family through the intensive care experience again. She went on by saying that she would never want life-support for herself, and asked if there was any way that she could ensure that wouldn't happen. I explained that there were, indeed, ways, and briefly reviewed the goals-of-care designation. I showed her the identifiable green-sleeve, goals-of-care binder, and how it could be used to ensure her management wishes would be clear to her caregivers. I then added that there was no rush at this stage to formalize the decision by filling out the document, and emphasized that it would be a good idea to discuss it with her husband and family first, particularly after more time had elapsed.

While we had been talking, I had noticed that she was wearing a gold cross necklace. After commenting on it, I asked if she had any church support. She replied by saying that they used to go to church, but had found attendance more difficult since the suicide. We discussed their other community supports, including friend groups and the be-reavement support group they had attended. Then I showed her my wooden cross that I wear underneath my shirt and tie. I mentioned briefly about my church involvement, and said, "Jesus knows about heartache, and I think He'd want to be present with you and comfort you in yours." She agreed and then sobbed some more. I passed her the Kleenex box and asked, "Would it help if I prayed with you right now?" She nodded in the affirmative, so I did, and prayed that she and her family might receive holy community comfort during this time of tragic loss. After the prayer, a Scripture came to me, which I wrote down on a prescription pad, and presented to her as she was leaving the clinic. It read, "The Lord is close to the broken-hearted and saves those who are

76

crushed in spirit" (Ps. 34:18).

In the wake of the devastation of suicide, it's important we recognize the suffering of the surviving family members and come alongside them in their time of grief. There's no denying the reality that suicide is a social tragedy. Suicide is the ultimate self-harm as it represents the wilful rejection of our identity as God's image bearers and an embrace of the fall as an end in itself with all its devastation and destruction. While we entrust the victims of suicide to a merciful God, all opportunity for healing, forgiveness, and reconciliation with family and friends are lost. Any suicide regret, which may have filled the person's dying mind during the final moments of neural activity, gets swallowed up by the silence of the grave. All is forever too late. Death retains its sting and cruelly celebrates its victory. So, we need to do our utmost to identify those at risk for suicide and do what we can to prevent suicide. In our present euthanasia-permissive society, this also means that we need to identify those patients in distress and despair who are more likely to request assisted suicide provision.

COUNTERING DESPAIR WITH DIGNITY

Fostering patient dignity and discovering ways for them to have meaningful experiences can be an effective means to diminish the existential despair they experience during illness and the dying process. In his book, *Man's Search for Meaning*, famed psychiatrist and Holocaust survivor Viktor Frankl discusses the problem of despair, and defines it as representing "suffering without meaning."[12] Many of Frankl's theories were developed from observations within the Auschwitz concentration camp during Nazi occupation. While facing similar levels of suffering, he noticed that some of his fellow inmates proved more resilient than others and more likely to survive. He discovered that those who had a reason to live were able to retain meaning in their suffering, and as a result, were less likely to succumb to despondency and death. Quoting Friedrich Nietzsche who said, "He who has a why to live for can bear almost any how," Frankl came to the conclusion that while all people suffered, despair occurred when meaning was stripped away from suffering.

To readily appreciate this concept, consider the pain that a woman experiences during childbirth as compared to the same level of pain experienced by someone with the advance of bone cancer. It's clear how the newborn baby can provide meaning and endurance for the suffering of the former, and how the bleak prospect of imminent death can rob the meaning and will to live in the latter. Frankl's Logotherapy approach was focussed on helping patients in the throes of existential suffering find meaning in their misery. This should be our goal, as well. To help offset the despair our patients may experience, our efforts should be aimed at helping them creatively discover meaning in their suffering. With meaning recovered, our prayer is that they will then be able to better face whatever suffering comes their way without resorting to requesting assisted suicide.

My first exposure to the spectre of existential suffering occurred while I was a medical student visiting my father in the hospital. During my clinical clerkship year, he suffered a massive stroke, surviving only by a narrow margin. Since it was before the era of thrombolytic therapy or interventional thrombectomy, which are routinely used in stroke management today, the brain damage he sustained was extensive and his neurological deficit was marked. In the twinkling of an eye, the once robust Naval Officer and dynamic preacher was reduced to a crippled old man in a wheelchair, with left side paralyzed and face drooping. After his prolonged recovery, he made several valiant attempts to return to some semblance of meaningful work. He tried his hand at writing, but found the concentration that it demanded too difficult. Drawing from his extensive theological knowledge, he attempted to lead Bible study once more, but because of his labile emotions and fatigability, he also found this too difficult. Determined not to give up, though, he even tried getting back into the pulpit. Although he did get the opportunity to deliver the Easter sermon, it was clear to all, himself especially, that his preaching days were over. And in his mind, the purpose of his life was gone. In his full-on perseverance, he met only discouragement and half successes. His loss of ability caused him to suffer greatly. Unable to find any meaning in his suffering, he developed significant depression and despair.

My father's anguish changed dramatically after a visit from one of his long-time friends and former parishioner. The friend was alarmed to see my father so downcast and blue. Recalling how his former pastor had been instrumental in his own life, the friend was determined not to leave my father in this sorry state. Looking around the room, he noticed a collection of family photos on my Dad's dresser, and pointing to them, said, "I know an important ministry for you! Look at all these precious faces of your family… they need you! You can help them by praying for each of them, every day…. God has given you this opportunity and the time to do it." The thought immediately resonated with my father, and before long, he was not only praying for each of his children and grand-children from his photo collection (myself included), but also a list of friends, and colleagues, as well as numerous hospital staff. Knowing that my father was a pastor and a "praying man," a number of nurses from his care facility started to visit him on a regular basis to receive prayer. He developed a vibrant intercessory prayer ministry, and continued this important work for the remainder of his life. The meaning he found through praying for others, and the dignity he experienced in the pro-cess, allowed him to endure and rise above his disabilities.

While there have been tremendous medical and technological advances in medicine since my father's stroke, in the critical realm of existential suffering, far less progress has been made. We can readily control physical symptoms these days, but when it comes to addressing the psychosocial and spiritual challenges patients are experiencing, we often flounder.[13] One promising clinical advance for reducing end-of-life existential suffering is referred to as *Dignity Therapy*. Developed by Canadian psychiatrist and palliative care specialist, Harvey Chochinov, this brief form of psychotherapy is aimed at improving the experiences of patients with end-stage illness.[14] Using a series of standard questions to promote meaningful personal reflection – including questions about their wishes, lessons learned, and how they want to be remembered – patients are interviewed by a trained counsellor, and their recorded responses are transcribed, edited, and provided for them as a lasting legacy document.[15] Originally designed for patients with low levels of distress, this simple tool has proven effective for patients with significant anxiety and depression, and has been found helpful to enhance the meaning, direction, and dignity of life for both patients and their families.[16] While I don't stick to the formal protocol, I have incorporated these types of questions in my routine conversations with patients who are in the throes of existential suffering. I've found that asking reflective questions of this nature can help a patient recover their self-worth, easily damaged by disease. As well, I make use of their responses to help me consider ways of recovering meaning in their lives, and means to offset the despair in their suffering.

THE CASE OF GRIEF AND A GUITAR

A case that illustrates the important role of dignity-promoting questions in helping to counter existential despair is of a patient who I managed on our cardiology ward. He was a rancher and former rodeo competitor in his mid-70s, who had a long history of ischemic heart disease. He had undergone two coronary artery bypass grafting surgeries in the past, as well as numerous percutaneous interventions, and now had inoperable coronary artery disease for which no further interventional solution was possible. I saw him after he had presented to hospital with crescendo angina requiring medical intensification. The nurses warned me that he was in a bad mood and complaining about his care. So, in order to have more time for our interaction, I decided to see him at the end of my rounds when I'd have more time to spend with him.

He looked his stated age or older, and was a large burly man with a gruff demeanour. I inquired about his symptom control and tried to build some rapport by asking about his rodeo days, to which he scoffed, "What's a city slicker like you interested in cowboy business for, any-ways?" Although I wasn't able to convince him that I'd formerly been a bronco rider, I did get a smile out of him when I clarified that my riding experience was during childhood and confined to the grocery store coin-operated variety of horses. As I was making some headway connecting with him, his lunch arrived, to which he whined, "Looks like a dog's breakfast" Then he started muttering about being better off dead and asked, "What's the good of medicines if I can't even care for my cattle without having to stop from chest pain? My ranch is my life. I'm totally useless like this. May as well have someone shoot me instead of having me carry on like this."

As he picked over his lunch, I asked him more about his background. He told me that he was widowed and had one grown son, who lived in town and had no interest in ranching. Now, because of his intractable symptoms, he was facing the reality of having to sell his land and give up his passion.

I asked him, "What were some of the most important parts of your life? When did you feel most alive?"

He paused, and then answered by saying it was riding his horses and taking part in one of the local rodeos. So, we talked about that for a while, and I mentioned how I enjoyed attending the Calgary Stampede over the years. Then, after washing his meatloaf down with some coffee, he mentioned that he'd also been part of a small-time country and blues band playing folk guitar. He smiled as he reminisced about those good ol' days when we used to "raise the roof on Saturdays and play at church on Sundays." As he said this, I remembered that I had a worship band practice myself the next evening, and would have my guitar with me during the day. So, I made a mental note to bring my guitar to the ward in an attempt to rekindle some of his old passion.

When I returned the next morning with my Martin acoustic in hand, and said he could use it till dinner, his eyes nearly popped out of his head. A large smile beamed across his face as I unpacked it from the case and placed it on his lap. "Play to your heart's content," I said. And sure enough, he did. He started off in a tentative way, but by the time our team had assembled to do ward rounds, we heard him strumming loud and clear and singing Johnny Cash-styled gospel tunes. Whether or not music can calm a savage beast I'm not sure, but in this case, it changed his demeanour and seemed to give him a new lease on life.

His son was so impressed with his father's improved mood that he restrung his old guitar and brought it in for him. The patient happily strummed away every day and at all times. So much so, in fact, that the nurses had to remind him about afternoon quiet time and sternly ring in the night-time curfew. There was no more talk about wanting to die. His passion for playing the guitar provided meaning in his present suffering and extinguished his desire to die.

This case reinforced in my mind that patients don't really want to die. They choose assisted suicide because in their present suffering, they see it as their only option. Desperate circumstances beget desperation. This would be the case for anyone who is contemplating suicide, and raises the conundrum of how we are supposed to separate them out. Who do we assist with their suicide and who should be prevented from killing themselves? By mandating that assisted suicide be included within Canadian healthcare services, the medical establishment has been placed in the impossible position of having to simultaneously reconcile both suicide prevention and suicide assistance. Where is the line demarcating the difference between suicide as a social tragedy and suicide as a medical obligation? Of course, any line drawn is an arbitrary one, moveable with time, and contrary to our biblical worldview.[17] As Christian healthcare professionals, therefore, our response should be to only and always prevent suicide. Regardless of the present MAID (Medical Assistance in Dying) laws in Canada, we must do our utmost to offset the request for its provision. Spending time with vulnerable patients and asking them dignity-promoting questions can go a long way to achieve this.

THE CASE OF HEART FAILURE AND LEGACY SUCCESS

Another example of countering existential suffering with dignity therapy was a case of heart failure in an elderly Dutch widow. She was in her early 80s and suffered from cardiac amyloidosis, which was causing pulmonary hypertension and peripheral edema necessitating admission to hospital. Although her chemotherapy for her amyloidosis had provided some temporary symptom benefits, she had now entered the end-stage of her disease and was being managed primarily with diuretic adjustments. Because of her poor heart function and marked leg swelling, she found any type of mobilization difficult and, as a result, had plunged into a reactive depression. During one of my interactions with her on our ward, she said that she was thinking about euthanasia and mentioned that she was aware of a number of her acquaintances who had done so in the Netherlands. In the hopes of brushing off the idea and redirecting her thoughts, I quipped, "Yes, thanks to Justin you can save airfare with *MAID* in Canada." Unwavering in her determination to die, she continued on the topic of euthanasia and asked me what my thoughts were on the subject. Still wanting to keep things light and downplay suicide as an end-of-life option, I used a modification of a Woody Allen line and said, "Even though we now have euthanasia in Canada, 'my relationship to death hasn't changed…. I'm still against it.'"

My answer made her smile, at least, which gave me the opportunity to ask her some reflective questions about her life's value, including her work and family. I inquired, "Are there specific things you want your family to remember about you?" to which she said there were a great deal of things. She mentioned that she had hoped to leave behind a legacy for her family in the form of collected memoirs from her WWII experiences. Although she had begun writing some time ago, she had found the task too large and complicated and abandoned her efforts. When I asked, "What are the most important roles you've had in life?" she said without hesitation, "being a grandmother," and then added, "And a great grandmother."

When I asked if she had any photos of her family, she showed me a group shot taken at a recent family reunion. Looking over the photo, I said, "There's your legacy right there. With all those grandchildren and great-grandchildren of yours, there must be someone who can help you pull your memoirs together. Why don't you invite some of them to be part of the project with you? After all, the company would be a nice change for you, and sometimes the process is as important as the product."

When I came to see her later that week, she was joined by two young ladies, one sorting papers and the other head down, and busy typing on a laptop. "No, time like the present, "she said to me with a youthful grin. "I've enlisted the help of my two great granddaughters here, and we're tackling my memoirs. There's more work to do than I thought. And I wouldn't want to miss out on a moment of it."

This case reinforces the fact that the request for assisted suicide represents a symptom of an unmet need. Our response is to prevent suicide ideation and the request for MAID. To do this, we need to take time to look behind the curtain of their request and get a better understanding as to the source of a patient's despair. Usually the request for assisted suicide stems from existential suffering related to: fear of dying, abandonment, loneliness, loss of control, futility, grief, guilt, duty, or some combination thereof. This is fertile ground for our priestly calling. As Christian healthcare professionals, we can speak to each of these issues. By asking reflective questions of the patient's life and experiences, we can help restore their dignity. And by creatively making use of their responses, we can explore ways to enhance the meaning in their lives, and offset the distress and despair in their suffering. Jesus calls us to abundant life, and this is what we want to offer our patients, even at the end of life.

CONCLUDING REMARKS

Healthcare is rife with suffering of many varieties, both physical and existential. One has to do little more than visit a busy downtown hospital emergency room, or walk through an overcrowded medical ward to appreciate this. Distress and despair are daily realities for both patients and providers, and need to be reconciled in some fashion. The biblical *fall* not only provides the foundation for our understanding of this challenged condition, but also an answer to why there is death and disease. It's our story. Each of us has been placed on the rising-action trajectory of the gospel narrative and given the option to either follow God in daily obedience or continue on in rebellion. How we respond to this moral matter will determine not only how we perceive our present circumstances – suffering and disease included – but also our final destiny. As Christian healthcare professionals, the spectre of suffering is a call to godly response. To keep faith in our practice, we need to protect ourselves from fatalistic thinking and hold tight to the cross of Christ, remembering that God has not abandoned us to our suffering, but meets us there. Patients also need to know that they are not abandoned during their times of travail. We are uniquely positioned to come alongside them and speak truth into their times of anguish, and hopefully cut the mounting of despair off at the pass. As Dr. Edward Pellegrino, the former Chairman of the President's Council on Bioethics said during my clinical clerkship at our hospital's Grand Rounds, "Physicians must never kill. Nothing is more fundamental or uncompromising." In order to negotiate such an uncompromising position, it's important to be involved early on in a patient's travail. Since request for suicide is a symptom of an unmet need, we can intervene by uncovering and addressing the underlying symptoms. By making use of dignity-fostering questions, we can help explore creative ways of addressing their existential suffering, and open a window to discovering meaning in their distress. In this way, it may be possible to prevent despair from taking an irreversible hold, and obviate their request for assisted suicide.

SUMMARY POINTS – THE FALL

1.   The doctrine of the fall provides the foundation for understanding the human condition and understanding our need for a personal saviour

2.   The cultural counter-narrative invokes chance as an explanation for reality

3.   If the doctrine of the fall is loosely held, so too, is the doctrine of salvation

4.   Our best protection from the spectre of despair is a well-defined theology of suffering focussed on the cross of Christ

5.   Prayer journaling can help to demonstrate God's intimate involvement in our personal lives and struggles

6.   Defining patient goals of care is an opportunity to address patient distress and discuss matters of faith

7.   The Holy Spirit can help to guide our patient interactions and prompt our witness of faith

8.   Request for euthanasia is a symptom of an unmet need

9.   Our Christian mandate is suicide prevention not assistance

QUESTIONS FOR REFLECTION AND DISCUSSION

1.   How does the doctrine of the fall assist you in coming to terms with the suffering in the world?

2.   What are your thoughts about the play of chance and its purported causative role in producing our reality?

3.   Have you experienced distress and despair in your own life?

4.   Do you have experience with the tragedy of suicide in your personal circle?

5.   What is your explanation for how God can be all-loving and powerful, yet allow suffering? How do you rationalize the occurrence of natural disasters? How do you give an explanation for moral evil or existence of disease and suffering in medicine? How do you defend the atrocities of the church? How would you defend God's wrath?

6.   What is your theology of suffering? Do you wear a cross?

7.   Have you experienced the hand of God in your life? Do you keep a prayer journal?

8.   What is your approach to defining patients' goals of care? Have you ever used this as an opportunity to address their existential suffering or discuss matters of faith?

9.   Do you ever receive a word, image, or nudge from the Holy Spirit? Has this ever happened in a clinical situation? How did you respond?

10. Have you prayed with a patient before? Why or why not?

11. How would you respond to a patient who asks for MAID?

12. Is there ever an indication for MAID?

CHAPTER NOTES

1. Mattos, E. McEwan S. *City of Death: Humanitarian Warriors in the Battle of Mosul.* Apollo River, 2018.

2. Statistics Canada: The 10 leading causes of death (2016).

3. Miller et al. Guns and Suicide in the United States. *New England Journal of Medicine* 2008; 359:989-991

4. Hsu, A.Y. *Grieving a Suicide: a loved one's search for comfort, answers, and hope.* IVP, 2017.

5. Leslie, K. *Medscape National Physician Burnout & Suicide Report 2020: The Generational Divide.* Jan. 15, 2020.

6. Edwin Arlington Robinson, "Richard Cory" published in *The Children of the Night.* 1897.

7. Garber, J. *God, Darwin, and the Problem of Evil.* Trafford Publishing, 2016.

8. Lutzer, E. *Where Was God? Answers to Tough Questions about God and Natural Disasters.* Tyndale House, 2006.

9. Larsen D. *The Company of the Creative: A Christian Reader's Guide to Great Literature and its Themes.* Kregel , 1999.

10. Lewis, C. S. *The World's Last Night.* Harper Collins, 1952.

11. Kaldjian, L.C., Erekson, Z.D., Haberle, T.H., et al. "Code status discussions and goals of care among hospitalised adults." *Journal of Medical Ethics 2009*; 35:338.

12. Frankl, V. *Man's Search for Meaning.* Beacon Press, 2006.

13. LeMay, K., Wilson, K.G. "Treatment of existential distress in life threatening illness: a review of manualized interventions." *Clinical Psychology Review* 2008; 28: 472–493

14. Chochinov, H.M. "Dignity-conserving care-a new model for palliative care: helping the patient feel valued." *JAMA* 2002; 287: 2253–2260

15. Chochinov, Harvey Max. *Dignity Therapy: Final Words for Final Days.* Oxford, 2012.

16. Martínez, M. "'Dignity therapy', a promising intervention in palliative care: A comprehensive systematic literature review." *Palliative Medicine.* 2017 Jun; 31(6): 492–509.

17. Alleyne, B., Van Maren, J. *A Guide to Discussing Assisted Suicide.* Life Cycle Books, 2017.

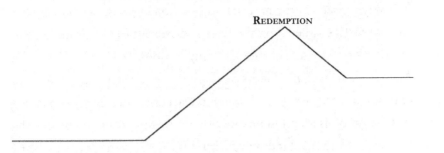

REDEMPTION

CHAPTER 3

SELF-RELIANCE AND SERVITUDE

"For the Lord is our judge, the Lord is our lawgiver, the Lord is our
King; it is He who will save us."

Isaiah 33:22

THE COST OF REJECTING SALVATION

The peak position or climax of the gospel contour represents God's
redemption of humankind by the death and resurrection of Jesus. Although God's plan of salvation for mankind is clearly woven throughout
the historical accounts and prophecies of the Old Testament, it was de-

finitively revealed in the ministry and passion of Jesus. Provided by His atoning sacrificial death on the cross and attested to by His miraculous resurrection, Jesus is our one and only Saviour. His name, *Yeshu'a*, in Aramaic translates as, "God saves." The apostle Peter emphasized this critical point to the rulers, elders, and teachers of the law by explaining that "salvation is found in no one else, for there is no other name under heaven given to mankind by which we must be saved" (Acts 4:12). By embodying the second Adam and acting as a penal substitute for God's wrath, Jesus conclusively brought an end to the fall's death grip on creation. The redemptive message for mankind is clear: it is God alone who saves, and not man. The heavy lifting is finished for us. Our role is simply to submit ourselves to God, repent of our rebellion, and believe. Through Jesus, there is the opportunity for the forgiveness of sins, freedom from bondage, healing of wounding, release from evil oppression, and the promise of eternal life. It's a breathtaking ultimate rescue. So, even though the effects of the fall continue to permeate our world today, they don't have the final word. As the apostle Paul said in the face of trial and tribulation, "We are hard pressed on every side, but not crushed; perplexed, but not in despair; persecuted but not abandoned; struck down, but not destroyed" (2 Cor. 4:8-9).

By contrast to this *Good News*, our contemporary culture arrogantly promotes a narrative of self-reliance. As a logical outworking of the popularized evolutionary worldview, the solutions to our problems are imagined to lie within the jurisdiction of self. Freed from the supposed shackles of God's plan and providence, our modern-day culture defiantly promotes the notion that our fitness alone is responsible for our survival and progress. Nelson Mandela captured this spirit of the times quite aptly when he quoted William Henley's *Invictus* saying, "I am the master of my fate and the captain of my destiny." Rather than a divine rescue from the troubles in our lives, the prevailing secular worldview

94

emphasizes a self-rescue. Instead of being encouraged to ask God for help, we are bombarded with self-help resources and prodded by motivational mantras such as, "do it your way," and "you can do anything you set your mind to." With the adoption of a salvation-through-works mindset, such thinking has even crept its way into the church. Despite our contemporary chorus music fixated on the message of salvation, when it comes down to the nitty-gritty challenges of daily life, even believers can end up relying more upon ourselves than upon God. As A.W. Tozer wryly observed, "Christians don't tell lies, they just go to church and sing them."

A self-help approach to life is doomed to failure. The Bible makes this clear. As stated in the Prophets, "My people have committed two sins: they have forsaken me, the spring of living water, and have dug their own cisterns, broken cisterns that cannot hold water" (Jer. 2:13). The burgeoning self-help sections of our bookstores attest to this painful reality: we simply can't do it on our own, but need help. While it may be possible for us to master a certain skill by viewing a ten-minute how-to YouTube video, we are certainly no masters of our lives, let alone our destiny. Captured in the lyrics of U2's gospel-lament, *I Still Haven't Found What I'm Looking For*, there remains a deep sense of longing and desire for something that this present age just can't satisfy. Referred to as our "incurable God-sickness" by Karl Barth, this existential discontent lies just beneath the surface of the brash exterior of every so-called self-made man. At the end of the day, despite our best efforts, we are left grabbing the air after some elusive dangling carrot – groping, grasping, clutching, but always left wanting. And the problem with a self-reliant approach to salvation is that it not only doesn't deliver, but it points us away from the personal, holy, and active God who does. In brief, self-reliance separates us from God. Distracted by the myriad of do-it-yourself options, it's easy to become blind to the outstretched arms of our Saviour and deaf to His knock to bring salvation into our lives. Without gospel redemption, we are left to our own impoverished devices to find some form of remedy for our deepest desires. However, despite our futile attempts to pull ourselves up by our own bootstraps, we remain mired in the mess of our human frailties. We can chant the Disney mantra to *believe in ourselves* ad nauseam, but the mirrored reflection of our honest gaze betrays our lack of self-confidence in this empty refrain. Sadly, these self-help attempts place us at risk for developing unhealthy attitudes and behaviours, and if left unchecked, can lead us down a descending path of self-destruction and servitude. As Scripture warns, "all you who light fires and provide yourselves with flaming torches, go, walk in the light of your fires and of the torches you have set ablaze. This is what you shall receive from my hand: you will lie down in torment" (Is. 50:11).

MEDICINE AND THE MONEY MASTER

Some healthcare practitioners deal with the frenetic stresses of the workplace by directing their self-reliance efforts towards money acquisition. They convince themselves that though the work is difficult, the monetary rewards are reasonable compensation, and will provide a sufficient solution to life's challenges. This was my error, too. Early on in my professional career, I found myself on the dreary treadmill of financial gain. It wasn't avarice. The desire for money wasn't on my mind when I entered medical school, or even when I began working in the hospital as a staff cardiologist. My honest goal was to help others and shine God's light into areas of need. But ever so slowly, and almost unperceptively, a transition occurred. My training years were long and hard, during which time I had to repeatedly defer life's pleasures. So, when my first pay cheques started coming in, I received them with a certain sense of self-entitlement, and considered my growing wealth as the well-deserved fruit of my labours. The more I made, the more I tended to spend, necessitating, of course, more money. So, in order to see more patients in less time, I improved efficiencies in my clinic, and chose certain tasks over others because of the financial reward. Over time, my energies were more and more focussed on ways of increasing my income and financial investments. As this occurred, my allegiance shifted away from God and towards a monetary idol. Although I was familiar with the apostle Paul's warning that "the love of money is a root of all kinds of evil," and that "Some people, eager for money, have wandered from the faith and pierced themselves with many griefs" (1 Tim. 6:10), I figured that I was different. After all, I rationalized, *God helps those who help themselves...* So, capitalizing on a housing boom in Edmonton, my wife and I developed a real estate business and set ourselves to the task of acquiring as many homes for rent as possible. And we were quite successful; so successful, in fact, that I'd probably have kept pushing us down that sorry path if it wasn't for the voice of the Holy Spirit awakening me to my misdirected efforts and growing self-reliance.

I was convicted of this waywardness quite unexpectedly. There was no dramatic prelude and I wasn't in church or near a confessional pew. Far from it, in fact. I was downstairs in our unfinished basement getting some exercise on my stationary bicycle. Earlier in the day, I had been reviewing my curriculum notes on the Ten Commandments in preparation for an upcoming Sunday school lesson. I was considering ways of presenting the Decalogue to the children in a more novel fashion. To foster some ideas, I read the commandments aloud, and then quietly started repeating them in cadence with my pedalling. When I got to the second commandment, "You shall have no other gods before me," and was thinking about some examples of idols that the children might relate to, money came to mind. Then I started hearing the refrain spoken not *by* me but *to* me. I felt immediately convicted of my own monetary idolatry. As I stopped pedalling, the warning of Jesus came to mind, "No one can serve two masters. Either you will hate the one and love the other, or you will be devoted to the one and despise the other. You cannot serve both God and money" (Matt. 6:24). Aware of my unhealthy attachment to money and the sinful place I'd allowed it to occupy in my life, I got off my bike and knelt beside the barbell bench to pray. As I confessed my sin, it become clear in my mind that I had allowed monetary self-reliance to become my means to salvation. I then recognized my need to recommit myself to Jesus, as Lord and Saviour of my life, which I did, right then and there, amid the cob-webbed cellar stud walls and surrounded by bags and boxes.

MONEY MATTERS

To protect ourselves from the financial idolatry related to self-reliance, it's important to exercise some caution when it comes to matters of money, including its earning, investing, and spending. God does not condemn wealth; He wants us to prosper. However, He also wants us to be aware that wealth can powerfully distract us from faith and lead us into the temptation of self-reliance. So, although there are unavoidable business considerations – in healthcare provision in general, and running a medical practice in particular – it's vital that we don't give the business end of medicine a life of its own and allow it to lead us astray. As William Osler rightly emphasized, "You are in this profession as a calling not as a business; as a calling which exacts from you at every turn self-sacrifice, devotion, love and tenderness to your fellow-men. Once you get down to a purely business level, your influence is gone and the true light of your life is dimmed. You must work in the missionary spirit, with a breadth of charity that raises you far above the petty jealousies of life."[1] Such words are important to keep this in mind, particularly as we meet with our accountants and financial advisors. Money matters, to be sure, but it doesn't matter most.

To help guard against the trap of idolizing money and having its acquisition and investment run our lives, it's worthwhile loosening our grip on the purse strings and intentionally giving generously. While we need to be good stewards of our resources, we should never be seen as stingy. Our financial sensibilities are not to align with the covetous Christmas Eve penny-pinching Ebenezer Scrooge-the-miser, but rather the reformed and magnanimous Christmas-morning Uncle Scrooge-the-spendthrift. As the apostle Paul says, "Whoever sows sparingly will also reap sparingly, and whoever sows generously will also reap generously. Each of you should give what you have decided in your heart to give, not reluctantly or under compulsion, for God loves a cheerful giver" (2 Cor. 9:6-7). And this is for good reason. Generosity is not only one of the fruits of the Spirit, it allows us to see material wealth for what it was intended to be – a tool for Kingdom work – rather than as an end in itself.

With generosity in mind, an effective spiritual discipline to consider is the commitment to regular tithing. The tithe is not only vital for the ongoing work of Christ's church, its regular practice fosters an attitude of thanksgiving for the blessings that we've received, and reminds us of our dependence on God for all good things. My wife and I have tried to tithe for most of our married life, and I recommend inculcating this spiritual discipline at the earliest stage possible. Like the attention to regular exercise, for example, the earlier tithing is developed, the easier it is to maintain. During my clinical clerkship in medical school, one of my mentors asked me what I did to keep fit. When I responded by saying I didn't have the time, he rebuked me with the comment, "If you can't find the time to exercise as a student, you'll never make it a priority when you're staff!" I would say something similar regarding the practice of tithing. The present is always a better time to establish this discipline than some nebulous future date. Our handling of money betrays our values. When we purchase an enormous estate home or some fully loaded luxury car, we communicate to the neighborhood the value we place on material possessions and their associated symbolic status. As we accrue wealth, it's important to keep Jesus' words in mind when He said, "For where your treasure is, there your heart will be also" (Matt. 6:21), and act accordingly.

Tithing is practicing what we're preaching. While the word "tithe" comes from an Old English root meaning "one tenth," we don't have to get nit-picky about amounts. The main principle behind tithing isn't so much a legalistic parting with a certain percentage of income, but a consistent spirit of generosity which demonstrates our unfailing love for Jesus and our concern for His bride, the Church. The patriarchs of the Old Testament originally set the tithing bar, with Abraham giving a tenth of his spoils of war to Melchizedek and Jacob promising God a tenth of everything granted him (Gen. 14:20; 28:22). Once codified in the Mosaic Law, the Israelites were commanded to give one tenth of their seed, fruit, and flocks to the Lord (Lev. 27:30-32) in order to support the Levites and their service in the temple (Num. 18:21-24). Although Scripture doesn't command us to give a tenth of our earnings today, as a spiritual discipline, this benchmark for giving can help protect us from permitting money to assume an unhealthy position in our lives, and from allowing self-reliance to dictate our modus operandi. So, rather than considering the ten percent as our gift to the church, my wife and I prefer to consider the ninety percent remaining as God's gift to us. Besides, the church desperately needs our support, particularly now in these hostile times. With the charitable status being placed on the chopping block by the government, and with dwindling numbers of parishioners, the church is significantly hindered in many of its ministries.

Our financial commitment can include not only monies for our local parish, but also support for the greater church, as well – the para-church – including Christian advocacy groups and Christian resource agencies, which together strengthen the church's inroads and influence in our society. Examples of para-church ministries worth supporting could include, Joe Boot's resource and equipping ministry of the Ezra Institute for Contemporary Christianity, John Carpay's Justice Center for Constitutional Freedoms, providing a legal voice for Christians under persecution, prolife advocacy organizations, such as the Canadian Center for Bioethical Reform, and Alberta's Wilberforce Project, as well as Alex Schadenberg's Euthanasia Prevention Coalition, to name a few. It's not that we need to restrict our giving to solely Christian ventures, but it's important that we prioritize faith-based groups, and the church, Christ's bride. By financially supporting both the local church, as well as biblically centered parachurch organizations, our hard-earned dollars can do more than we could ask or imagine.

PROTECTION FROM SELF-IDOLATRY

As healthcare professionals immersed in the medical culture of pseudo-salvation, we need to consciously protect ourselves from the lure of self-reliance. I've learned this the hard way, and have come to appreciate that the first and foremost step to guard ourselves against this variety of self-idolatry is ensuring that we are in proper relationship with God. This entails both considering who God is rightly, and fostering an intimate relationship with Him. In our culture of all things informal, from our casual attire and off-the-cuff, coarse comments, to our unceremonious behaviours, it's a short step to consider God in some lesser way as well, Jesus our buddy. But this is hardly a biblical understanding of

God. The Scriptures make clear that "As the heavens are higher than the earth, so are His ways higher than our ways and His thoughts higher than our thoughts" (Isa. 55:9). While God certainly loves us unconditionally and is personal and directly accessible to each of us, He can't be reduced to some mini Jesus-in-the-pocket that we can pull out at our pleasing. There is a critical creature/Creator distinction that we must not lose sight of, nor forget that we are the creature part, and that God is the all-powerful, all-knowing, and ever-present Creator of the universe part, and not the other way around. So, we need to know our place in the vast configuration of things. As Evelyn Underhill writes, "any spiritual view which focusses attention on ourselves, and puts the human creature with its small ideas and adventures in the centre foreground, is dangerous till we recognise its absurdity."[2]

To consider God rightly, then, we would do well to dust off the ancient biblical expression, *Fear of the Lord*, and give it due attention. This bound phrase (which is perhaps better written, Fear-of-the-Lord) appears frequently throughout the Old Testament, and refers not only to a deep respect and knee-knocking reverence for God, but also implies a posture of submission and willing obedience on our part. As Eugene Petersen wisely observed, "Its function as a single word cannot be understood by taking it apart and then adding up the meanings of the part... It is the stock biblical phrase for the way of life that is lived responsively and appropriately before who God is, who he is as Father, Son and Holy Spirit."[3]

Coming before God in this way, and trusting in Him with our whole life, allows for a special form of intimacy to develop. This understanding was alluded to by King David when he said, "The Lord confides in those who fear him" (Ps. 25:14) and is ours to cherish if we so choose.

To combat Messiah-complex sort of thinking, we need to be reminded of our limitations and God's limitlessness. To better foster an intimate relationship with our awesome God, I begin each day with a brief time of solitude and confessional prayer. Henri Nouwen, who regularly devoted an entire hour each morning to prayer, said, "If we really believe not only that God exists, but also that he is actively present in our lives – healing, teaching, and guiding – we need to set aside a time and space to give him our undivided attention."[4] While I don't have the luxury of taking a full hour for my devotional time, or even a quarter of that, I make it a priority to quiet myself before the Lord every morning during my breakfast routine. Using my devotional, A *Guide to Prayer for Ministers and Other Servants*,[5] as a resource text, my morning reflection begins as I put the kettle for tea on to boil. Organized around weekly devotional themes, the format of this guide is ideal for habitual reflection and includes a prayer of invocation, a Psalm for the week, a daily Scripture reading, as well as some assorted readings. Depending on the length of Scripture for the day, I can usually get to the reflected reading portion by the time my tea is steeped. Then, after I've eaten, I sit quietly in God's presence for a quiet moment and enter into a focussed time of listening prayer. As Helmut Thielicke said, "To work without praying and without listening means only to grow and spread oneself upward, without striking roots and without an equivalent in the earth."[6] So, in a desire to deepen my roots in the Lord, I ask God if there is any area of my life which He would like to bring to my attention, in which I've chosen self-reliance over his salvation, and I quietly listen. It doesn't take long. Usually within brief moments, a picture or memory comes to mind, providing an opportunity for me to pray into dark areas of my inner life and develop greater intimacy with God. I close my time of devotion by confessing the Sinner's Prayer, "Lord Jesus Christ, Son of God, have mercy on me, a sinner," and then set off for work, with "eyes fixed on Jesus the author and perfecter of our faith" (Heb. 12:2).

MISSION MATTERS

Over the years, I've had the opportunity to take part in a variety of outreach Christian missions, which have functioned as poignant reminders of my dependence on God, and taught me the invaluable lesson of trusting in God's provision. Working in resource-poor settings distant from our diagnostic toys and familiar disease patterns not only improves our clinical skills and broadens our differential diagnoses, it forces us to rely more upon God and less upon ourselves. One such formative experience occurred early in my training as a cardiology resident, during the Rwandan Genocide of 1994. Referred to by President Clinton as "the world's worst humanitarian crisis in a generation," the cholera outbreak grabbed the headlines, and captured my imagination. Keen to help, I joined a small Canadian medical contingent financially supported and commissioned by our local church. Our mission was to work alongside the local relief efforts in the border town of Goma, to provide medical assistance to the Hutu exiles in former Zaire (today's Democratic Republic of Congo). So, our team of doctors and nurses set off with a congregational blessing, a spirit of charity, and bags brimming with medical supplies and goodwill provisions.

When we arrived, however, things weren't as we had expected. To our surprise and dismay, we discovered that our on-ground personnel were no longer available to transport us to the refugee camps, and that our medical connections – forged over months of overseas correspondence – had vaporized. The team was naturally disappointed. We had taken time out of our work and training, travelled across the world with needed medical equipment and expertise (at significant expense), but found ourselves unable to be meaningfully involved. It was a frustrating all-dressed-up-but-no-place-to-go predicament. However, before we could get too far down the dark spiral of self-pity, an elderly pastor from a local church met with us. He had a calm demeanor, and listened

104

patiently as we described our dilemma. Then, rather than joining our chorus of woe and distress, he focussed our attention onto what he felt was the real issue at hand – trusting in God's provision. He read from the book of Genesis detailing Abraham's testing, and how God had provided a ram to sacrifice in place of Isaac. He used this Scripture as a grounding text for us to consider as he encouraged us, despite our bleak present circumstances, to trust in God's provision to remedy our situation. Then he prayed over each of us, appealing to God by the holy moniker, *Jehovah-Jireh*, or "God will provide."

Although I appreciated his wise perspective and heartfelt prayer, I didn't hold much stock in such "wishful thinking," as I perceived it. So, since I had pretty much abandoned any hopes of medical service during our stay, I used my time to explore the bustling markets and to take long walks along the neighboring steep grassy hills bordering the city. One morning, while overlooking Lake Kivu from a steep perch, I prayed to God and confessed my lack of trust in Him. I asked that opportunities for useful involvement might be provided to rescue our stalled mission. And despite my earlier incredulity, my prayer was answered, and then some. The adage, *be careful for what you pray for* rang true for me that day. Not only were medical connections forged for our team to work in the local hospital, but transportation to a refugee clinic in one of the five-cholera ravaged camps was also made possible.

After spending a couple of weeks doing hospital rounds, our team finally set off for the refugee camp. We had to make our way across black volcanic ridges, navigating pothole-riddled muddy roads from the North Kivu capital of Goma to the sprawling Kibumba refugee camp, where nearly half a million refugees sought temporary shelter. Crammed tightly into the back of the 4-wheel drive, and still a fair distance from our destination, I could spy the vast array of UN-supplied blue tents of the camp, which dotted the misty jungle hills for miles. As we arrived at the camp entrance, a multitude of faces received us with blank stares, amid a chaos of cooking fire smoke, yelling, and confusion. The clinic tent was located deep in the center of the camp, necessitating that we wind along steep muddy trails to an upper plateau. The crowd ahead slowly separated to allow us passage, and then closed behind us again, swallowing our vehicle in a mass of human suffering.

When we pulled up to the clinic, we saw a staggering number of patients lined up waiting for assessment, many of whom, we were told, had camped through the night to keep their place in the queue. The medical supplies were basic to our needs and included fresh water, bandages and splints, and a limited assortment of antibiotics and analgesics. I was armed with my trusty Littmann stethoscope and Welch Allyn diagnostic set, as well as a tattered copy of the Gideon Bible, complete with bookmarked passages and some Swahili phrases. The nurses from our team helped triage patients, directing the sicker ones my way. "God help me," I remember muttering as I laid out our supplies. And then just as I was preparing to examine the first of the refugees, a remarkable warm feeling came over me, and the words, "you help me," came to mind. I shivered, and in reflex response replied aloud, "Yes Lord. Here am I," and rolled up my sleeves to the tasks at hand.

Although the medicine I practiced in the refugee camp was of the most basic variety, God's presence was palpable to me and galvanized in my mind that He is trustworthy and will provide. The experience taught me that as we move outside of our comfort zones, the Holy Spirit draws nearer. In keeping with the inspirational quote that "those who leave everything in God's hand will eventually see God's hand in everything," I have found that during the challenging moments in the mission field, when I am pushed beyond my rote and routine, I become more acutely aware of the Holy Spirit's presence and His active involvement in my life. It's as if our discomfort pries our fingers from the rope of self-reliance and frees our hands to receive what God wishes to bestow. When our hearts are softened in this way, our focus is naturally drawn away from the narrow pragmatic delivery of technical expertise, and directed more towards a broader relational provision of relief and comfort. As we engage in the mission field – local or abroad – we become more likely to see patients as "fellow travellers to the grave and not another race of creatures bound on other journeys,"[7] and see ourselves – our kind words and reassuring touch – as the medicine.

Another illustrative example of this was when I was more recently in Cameroon, assisting in medical provision at a remote Baptist hospital, and helping to establish an internal medicine residency teaching program. Facilitating EKG reading and demonstrating the utility of hand-held ultrasound was my main focus. But while I was there, I was also given the duty of rounding on the medical ward. It was a Colonial-styled single-room ward, crowded to capacity, with a double row of sick patients on gurneys, surrounded by their accompanying family members. I felt quite overwhelmed seeing patient after patient suffering from tropical diseases of every sort, with only the very occasional heart issue that rang any familiar bells. However, I had no difficulty in recognizing one particular disease pattern well-represented on the ward – end-stage HIV. Reminiscent of my medical school training experiences, I saw numerous cases of severe wasting secondary to disseminated AIDS in Cameroon. Unable to afford the subsidized anti-retroviral therapy or distrustful of its western origin, there were large numbers of patients dying a similar death to those I cared for as a clinical clerk in Vancouver back in the '80s.

One such patient, a middle-aged cachectic gentleman, was dutifully attended to by his two teenage sons, similar in age to my own boys. "What on earth can I possibly do for this one?" I thought to myself,

107

as I listened to the hospitalist relay the history. And then words from Matthew immediately came to mind, "Whatever you do for one of the least of these, you do for me (Matt. 25:40). So, I sat down beside the dying patient, put a cold cloth on his forehead, and demonstrated for his sons how they could comfort their father by keeping his mouth and lips moist using an oral sponge swab and cup of water. Then, through the help of two sets of translators (one translating from my English to French, and the second translating from French to their local dialect), I communicated the gravity of the situation to the boys, which they seemed to understand. With the two gathered closely around, I had the translators repeat my reading of Psalm 23 and prayers of solace over the patient. The next day, there were additional family members accompanying the teens at the patient's bedside. Despite his deteriorating condition, the family members seemed very pleased with the care he was receiving. They came up to me, each in turn, shook my hand, and warmly expressed their thanks for "doing so much."

Although at the time I didn't feel that I had done much at all, I've since come to realize that there is something therapeutic about spending time with patients. The comfort I had offered the dying man and his family did little to stave off his imminent death, but as it turned out, was the remedy that more fully met their needs. For this reason, I highly recommend outreach Christian mission involvement for trainees and post-graduates alike, from every discipline of healthcare. Working with fellow brothers and sisters in Christ grows us spiritually, and provides opportunities to learn and model Christian discipleship in the provision of healthcare. I've gained confidence from these experiences to witness my faith to others and share the gospel's lifesaving message. As Oswald Chambers emphasized, "the one great reason under all missionary enterprise is not the elevation of the people, nor their education, nor their needs, but first and foremost the command of Jesus Christ."[8]

So, while good works may be undertaken by a variety of charitable organizations, as Christian practitioners, our primary calling in the mission field is to follow the Great Commission.

DIVINIZATION OF MEDICINE

The razzle and dazzle of modern medicine feeds into the self-reliance craze of our culture, and can distract even Christian practitioners and patients from turning to God during times of trouble. The significant technological breakthroughs enjoyed in modern medicine have been wonderful and are important to mark and celebrate, but they have their snare. Our medical advances have given rise to an over-reliance on healthcare as a solution to all our problems. With the exception of end-stage disease states, no longer are the provision of comfort or relief of pain adequate goals of care. Rather, nothing short of complete cure seems acceptable. In a real sense, healthcare has become the religion of our time, with health practitioners its designated priests.

This divinization of healthcare is reminiscent of medical practice in the polytheistic Greco-Roman era.[9] While homage is often paid to the classic figures of Hippocrates, Aristotle, and Galen, our contemporary medicine holds little resemblance to their pagan practices. Unlike our current research-based medical practice, which was founded on the Christian worldview, their medical art relied heavily upon metaphysical speculation and was very much interwoven with the occult. Physicians of antiquity were seen as agents representing the demi-gods of healing, and were tasked to command or manipulate nature by use of secret knowledge and skill. And without the personal knowledge of a loving God, as revealed in Scripture, a patient's singular hope at that time was understood to be through medicine's mediated influence of nature. Although the incantations and recipes may have changed since those dark days of

Hippocrates and the humoral theory, there is a definite overlap between patients of antiquity and present time in terms of their medical-reliance mindset. Our society is steeped in a self-help culture. Having exhausted their own limited supply of do-it-yourself resources, patients can easily be drawn to the awe and sparkle of medicine to provide a remedy for their aches and pains, and even deeper issues, as well. The current rash of television medical dramas have popularized this go-to strategy considerably. In such programing, the medical doctors are portrayed as flesh and blood heroes of our times, and the medicine profiled is nothing less than miraculous. It should come as no surprise, then, that some of our patients hold up unrealistic expectations of medicine.

So, in addition to taking intentional steps to safeguard ourselves as medical practitioners from the lure of self-reliance in medicine, we need to protect our patients, as well, from the pseudo-salvation of healthcare and the idolatry of medicine. Many of my patients hold to this sort of naïve misunderstanding of healthcare. Demanding much, and expecting more, they are often in search of some procedure or pill that will provide a solution to their troubles. One such patient of mine who exemplified this salvation strategy was a middle-aged woman who worked as a hospital unit clerk. I was asked to see her to investigate her exertional dyspnea. Because of her numerous cardiovascular risk factors, her family physician was concerned that her symptoms might reflect underlying heart disease.

When I knocked on the clinic door and entered the room she was just finishing a chocolate bar, and as she was wiping her mouth, she sheepishly said, "no time for *breckie* this morning... but it's only 100 calories."

I smiled and shook her hand, replying, "Yes, I guess that's why Mom always called it the most important meal... leads us not into temptation."

After inquiring about her symptoms and examining her, I felt that even though she had mild hypertension and glucose intolerance that her symptoms weren't anything sinister, and most likely related to deconditioning, amplified by her obesity. When I breached the topic of body weight and physical activity with her, she said defensively that she was unable to exercise because of her knee arthritis. Then in a more animated tone she exclaimed, "That's why I want to have an angiogram. I need to have my heart checked out to make sure I'm okay for my surgeries."

"Surgeries?" I queried with surprise. "Your family physician didn't mention anything to me about a pre-operative consultation. What surgeries are you referring to?"

"Knee surgery, of course," she replied impatiently, "and bariatric surgery. Once I get these knees done and my stomach stapled, I'll be able to get back to my normal body weight and be more active. My biggest problem is having to wait for all these doctors' appointments and tests to get booked. I just want to get on with my life. Why do these things have to take so long?"

"Yes," I said in agreement, as I invited her to come down from the examination bed and sit on a more comfortable chair. "Our healthcare system can be a bit frustrating, particularly when we're having to wait." And then I pondered to myself… "Where to begin?"

When we have patient interactions of this sort, it's important to practice patient-*centered* medicine and resist patient-*directed* medicine. It's not necessarily in a patient's best interest – and certainly not good medicine – when we simply follow patient requests.[10] This includes addressing the patient's root issues and not getting sidetracked by some rabbit-hole test result or latest study. So, rather than endorsing her surgical salvation mindset, and simply booking her for an angiogram, which would've taken only a few minutes, I chose instead a more time-consuming path. Instead of paper pusher, I took on the more satisfying role of patient educator, and reviewed the risks and benefits of her desired interventions, as well as their merits and limitations. Although this takes more time and effort, teaching is an integral element of our priestly calling. The term, doctor, in Latin means "teacher," from *docere* ("to teach"). In the early church, the moniker, *doctor*, was applied to teachers of Christian doctrine, and was only more recently used by the medical profession to denote physician.[11] So, as Christian healthcare professionals, we have a teaching mandate, and should look for teaching opportunities in our clinical interactions.

As part of our discussion, then, I made a concerted effort to steer her away from the idolatry of medicine, and towards a broader understanding of wellbeing. I tried to lay out some practical ways in which she could be an active participant in improving her health. In particular, I reviewed the long-term strategy of weight control and how intermittent fasting can be an effective way to achieve this.[12] As well, I detailed the key elements of a healthy diet, emphasizing the value of choosing whole foods and natural fats with some examples, as well as the importance of avoiding sugar and refined grains with some other examples. I explained how glucose activates our neural reward pleasure pathway causing the neurotransmitter, dopamine, to be released, which in turn can lead to food addiction.[13]

At that point she admitted to having a sweet tooth and being "a stress eater." She confessed to often indulging in confections through the day and dessert items in the evening. So, I suggested that a good place for her to start would be to eliminate all processed simple sugars from her cupboards at home with an "out of sight, out of mind" type of approach. Then, when I asked her about her sources of stress, she suddenly burst out in tears, and explained how she and her husband of 27 years were recently separated and considering divorce.

"That sounds really difficult," I empathized, as I passed her some tissue. "Who do you have around you for support? Any family in town… friend groups… do you belong to a church family?"

After I listened for a while, I suggested that salvaging her marriage would be a priority over embarking on the surgeries she had mentioned. I agreed to make arrangements for her to see our dietician, and encouraged her to reach out to her support network and engage the involvement of a marriage counselor.

Medicine is important, but it can't save us. Unless we understand healthcare as an aspect of God's greater healing and redemptive work in history, medicine can easily take on a life of its own and become a source of idolatry. We need to guard ourselves and our patients against divinizing medicine. As healthcare professionals, we may have useful skills and important knowledge, but we are not medical messiahs. Patients need to know that there are limitations to what we can do and to what modern medicine can offer. A frank patient-centered approach as illustrated can be helpful to address these realities. Such a discussion may take more time than simply going along with a patient's wishes for investigation or treatment, but might be instrumental in pointing them towards the One who can save.

ADDICTION MEDICINE

When people all-out reject God's message of salvation, the option of self-help is commonly chosen. And it's a short step from self-help to self-medicate. As individuals get trapped in the lie of self-sufficiency, they run the risk of developing unhealthy behaviours, which can lead to addiction and self-harm. Once addictive drugs enter the scene, then dependence, compulsive behaviour, tolerance, and a downward spiral of destruction can easily ensue. Alcohol and drug addiction are rampant in our society, and I see a great deal of their aftermath at the downtown hospital where I practice. Over the past few years, we've had a rash of Fentanyl overdoses, with story after story of senseless fatalities and shattered lives. Activating the same naturally-existing neural pathway as sex and food, addictive drugs cause the release of the neurotransmitter, dopamine, into the synaptic junctions of our brain's reward circuit. However, unlike food and sexual intercourse, they have the capacity to release far more dopamine, and at a much faster rate, resulting in a significantly higher addictive potential. For these reasons, drug addictions can be exceedingly challenging to treat.[14]

Most of my involvement in this area of medical intervention has been with patients battling nicotine addiction in my smoking cessation clinic. There I listen to patients' quit-attempt stories and discuss various options available to help them gain control over their *cancer stick* enslavement. Practicing in the inner city, however, I'm also in close proximity to the challenges of the street, and am regularly involved in the care of patients who abuse intravenous drugs. As such, I'm regularly asked to see patients when they present with fever of undetermined origin, to see if they might have heart valve involvement with their systemic infection.

One of my patients was a 28-year old aboriginal intravenous drug user, who had bounced from shelter to shelter over the years, and lived, for the most part, on the streets of downtown Edmonton. She had had numerous past hospital admissions with intoxication and various infections, and had exhausted several of our counselors and social workers. She had even been reviewed by our specialized Addiction Recovery and Community Health Team (ARCH), and refused their assistance. Notwithstanding, and despite the numerous needle exchange program locations in the downtown, and our hospital-based supervised consumption site, she once again resurfaced with drug withdrawal complicated by sepsis. When I examined her on this occasion, she had clinical findings of severe tricuspid valve insufficiency, as indicated by her distended neck veins and pulsatile liver. So, I prepared to perform a transesophageal echocardiogram to assess her heart valves for the possibility of endocardial vegetations.

After I explained the procedure to her and obtained informed consent, I began to slowly administer a combination of intravenous Fentanyl and Midazolam to produce a temporary conscious sedation, in order to perform the study. While doing so, I noticed that she was wearing a cross necklace and, commenting on how nice it looked, asked if she attended church.

"No," she replied curtly. "My grandmother gave it to me. She goes to Sacred Heart once in a while."

"Oh yes, that's just a few blocks away, isn't it? It's the First Nation's parish, right?" I asked, hoping to build on a connection. "I've been told that their liturgy uses native drums and sweet grass, and the like."

"I wouldn't know," she replied flatly. "It sounds stupid."

"Well, your grandmother doesn't think so," I countered. "And neither do I. Have a look at my mine," I said, as I displayed the leather cord with dangling wooden cross from under my shirt.

"Oh, why do you wear a cross? Are you afraid of vampires or something?" she teased.

"Not scared of monsters, so much," I answered with a smile. "But I am concerned about thinking I need to solve all the world's problems myself. The cross is important because it reminds me that I don't have to, and that Jesus knows about our pain and problems and wants to save us from ourselves."

Then, as she started to doze off, I proceeded with the test. However, as I was gently inserting the probe into her mouth, she suddenly clamped down hard with her teeth, nearly taking off my index finger. I attempted again (this time even more cautiously), and again she clamped down. I tried to encourage her cooperation, but the more I appealed, the more she resisted. Since there was little point in trying to reason with her any further, I called off the procedure.

As I was putting away the probe and removing my gloves, she smiled and said mockingly, "I got what I wanted. Thanks for the drugs, Holy Joe. They're real good." Then she drifted off into the drug-induced bliss that was of my own making.

Addiction is ugly business. We can do a great deal in modern medicine, but there are definite limitations, particularly in the area of addiction medicine. Not all of my addiction cases are quite as frustrating as this one, but a key generalizable point to emphasize is that we shouldn't give up on people, including the ones that seem beyond hope. Our role is to come alongside patients in their illnesses and suffering. We need to attempt to shine God's light into their lives, even if it doesn't seem to make any difference at the time. In this, of course, we have certain responsibilities, but we don't have ultimate responsibility. That is God's domain and His alone. Finally, we can do our best, and no more.

This case also illustrates the limited benefit of a harm reduction strategy. Supervised injection sites for intravenous drug use have certainly been shown to reduce mortality and infection transmission, including HIV transmission, but care must be taken to ensure that we don't simply enable people in their addictive behaviours.[15] While mortality reduction is an important step, it shouldn't be our endgame objective. Our goal in medicine is not simply the reduction of harm, but the optimization of health for body and soul. Saving lives and reducing harm need to be part of a broader strategy to free patients from the enslavement of addiction. We can use such facilities as an opportunity to develop relational connections with those who suffer from addiction, and by way of relationship, steadily direct them towards health. So, if we are to develop and fund safe-injection sites, which is a controversy in and of itself that needs to be debated and discerned, it certainly needs to be with this greater human flourishing objective in mind.

THE CASE OF RECONCILIATION AND REHAB

I had another patient who also struggled with addiction, but who, by contrast, in the end heeded my counsel. He had recently presented to hospital with a large heart attack and was admitted to the cardiology ward which I was supervising. He was HIV positive, and smoked a combination of tobacco, as well as both recreational and medicinal marijuana. Although he was only in his late 40s, he was found to have extensive coronary artery disease with left main involvement, for which bypass surgery was the only real interventional option. But, unfortunately, he would have nothing of it. When the nurse explained to me that he was refusing surgery and was planning to leave, I made a beeline to his room to discuss matters. When I arrived, I found his room empty, and figured I was too late.

"He hasn't left just yet," the nurse reassured me. "He's just gone outside for another smoke."

Since there were no pressing issues on the ward, I decided to track him down and walked out to the "smoker's courtyard" (officially a non-smoking area, which had been overtaken by those addicted to nicotine). I saw a smoker sitting alone on one of the benches wearing a hospital gown with IV pole in tow. Surmising it was my patient, I introduced myself, and sat down next to him. I opened with some comments about the weather, and gently asked him some questions about how things were going and what his plans were. As we talked, it became clear that his refusal for surgery and threat to leave the hospital were entirely fear-based responses. This present admission was his very first time in hospital, and he was petrified. When he asked me questions about the surgical procedure, I explained them to him, but added that he was the

117

boss, and no one was going to force him to have surgery. I underscored that surgery was his best option, particularly if he wanted to carry on with the plans he had mentioned to me.

Fortunately for his sake, he agreed to stay. So, I put his name back on the in-patient surgical waiting list, and every morning after my rounds, I'd spend some extra time with him, listening to his story and offering him some perspective. He shared with me about his loneliness and his estrangement from his family, on the account of his sexual orientation. I encouraged him to connect with them, nonetheless, and at least inform them of his admission to hospital and pending operation. Still somewhat fearful, he asked me about smoking cessation and if marijuana was safer than cigarettes. And although I could sense his disappointment with my answers – that marijuana was equally as harmful as tobacco, concerning cardiovascular effects in whatever form consumed, smoked, vaped, edible, or otherwise; and that quitting both tobacco and cannabis would be critical for his health – he wasn't overly surprised. On the day before he was transported to our surgical site, his family had gathered in his room. It was good medicine to see this type of reconciliation take place. And when I saw him in follow-up some months later, he had quit smoking (marijuana included) and had joined a local gym, "to stay healthy and on the right side of the *grass*," as he put it.

BEHAVIOURAL ADDICTION

One form of addiction that is particularly challenging to treat is the area of behavioural addictions, such as gambling and Internet pornography. Like narcotic drugs, these behaviours activate our brains' pleasure pathway and, mediated by dopamine release into the reward circuit, can produce an equally powerful addiction. In fact, Internet pornography can produce a sustained level of dopamine release that no drug can match. This is in part because of the unlimited novelty of online images available to the viewer, where every click of the mouse produces yet another neurotransmitter surge flooding the reward circuit and maintaining the heightened dopamine levels. Not surprisingly, Internet pornography has been likened to the new crack cocaine.[16] In some respects it's even worse. With substance abuse addiction, we at least have proven effective therapies to help reduce withdrawal symptoms: the long-acting opioid, Methadone, for example, can act as a drug substitute and provide a more graduated detoxification for patients with opiate addiction. Unfortunately, the pharmacological arsenal for behavioural addictions, including pornography addiction, is pretty bare. Counseling programs, behavioural modification strategies, and mindfulness-based interventions constitute the mainstay of medical interventions, and are time-consuming and not always particularly successful.

While patients aren't sent to me for the management of behavioural addictions, the trouble does surface on occasion. One such patient, who was sent to me for assessment of palpitations, is an example, and illustrative of behaviour addiction challenge. He was in his late 30s and worked as a computer programmer at the university. He was well-kept and fit-appearing, and married with two young children. He had heard that I was a Christian physician, so he comfortably shared with me that he attended church, and was quite active in both the music and children's ministries. In short, he was a *together* fellow, and quite unlike most of my other patients who seem to have more obvious struggles. On discussing his symptoms, he described episodes where he felt that his heart was racing, usually at night, and for no reason he could pinpoint. It sometimes interrupted his sleep, forcing him to retreat to another bed so as not to awaken his wife. He mentioned that the episodes were causing him considerable anxiety and that his resultant mood was negatively impacting the time with his children. When I asked about caffeine consumption and life stressors, he admitted to having only two cups of coffee a day and mentioned some work-related issues, but nothing of any consequence.

His echocardiogram showed a structurally-normal heart, and his 24-hour Holter monitor had recently been completed, and was totally benign. It showed regular heart rhythm with only very occasional extra heart beats. So, without much to grab onto for a diagnosis, I asked him what he thought might be causing his symptoms. He blushed, looked down at his feet, and then reluctantly confessed to frequent use of Internet pornography with masturbation, and was wondering if this might be the cause and affecting his health.

"Nothing that will directly harm your heart," I reassured him, "but a great deal that could harm your mind and soul, not to mention your relationships, particularly with your wife. Internet pornography can lead to quite a serious form of addiction." After a pause, I asked him point-blank, "Do you want to quit?"

"More than anything else in the world," he said, now with his eyes tearing up.

"Then the first order of business," I emphasized, "is getting away from Internet pornography. To do so you will likely need to relinquish your right to computer privacy. So, at least for the time being, limit your Internet use to only public places, like coffee shops, the cafeteria, your crowded office, and your kitchen at home. I've raised three boys, and know this from experience. Only by dissociating the Internet from pornography can you hope to get a handle on the monster of pornography addiction."

I went on to describe the physiologic basis for Internet pornography addiction and the structural neurologic consequences that can ensue. I prepared him for the battle he was facing by saying how it would take some weeks, if not months, for those neurocircuitry changes to revert towards normal, and for the desires to diminish. I outlined the value of having an accountability partner with whom he could have regular check-ins, like a friend from church, and I also mentioned a couple of helpful resources for him to check out.[17,18] To give him a biblical handhold for the fight, I wrote him a Scripture script with helpful verses to ingrain in his mind.

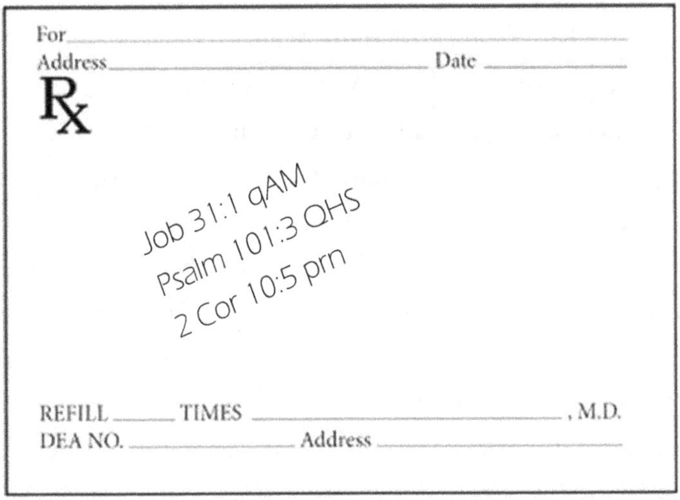

Figure 1. Scripture Script for Pornography Addiction

Finally, I mentioned the need to replace his desires for pornography with an alternate affection. I encouraged him to become more immersed in reading the Word and pour energy into his marriage, and plan some intentional dates with his wife. I concluded our time together by praying over him saying, "To him who is able to keep you from stumbling and to present you before his glorious presence without fault and with great joy" (Jude 24).

Pornography addiction is pervasive in our society. It's estimated that one third of our entire Internet bandwidth is devoted to pornography, with upwards of eighty percent of men and thirty percent of women viewing it monthly.[19] Church attendees or members, and even church leadership are not exempt. Over half of Christian pastors recently interviewed admitted to regular pornography consumption.[20] It's been said that every man who knocks at the door of a brothel is actually looking for God. Similarly, when people click their mouse over a porn site, they betray a longing for something more: a certain remedy or solution to an inner emptiness or some form of salvation, however twisted and depraved. Addictions in general, and pornography addiction in particular, are dreadfully harmful for both those bound to them, as well as those in their circle, and society at large. As Mary Anne Layden, director of the Sexual Trauma and Psychopathology Program at the University of Pennsylvania has attested, pornography degrades women, trivializes sexual assault, and fuels rape culture.[21] Christian healthcare professionals need to be aware of the magnitude of these demonic challenges and reach out in care and compassion to those caught in the clutches of pornography addiction, redirecting them towards gospel redemption. As the apostle John proclaims, "So if the Son sets you free, you will be free indeed" (John 8:36). Only with Christ's salvation can there be true freedom, human flourishing, and health in its fullest.

CONCLUDING REMARKS

The spirit of self-reliance is pervasive in medical culture. Healthcare provision is very much a nose-to-the-grindstone type of vocation. In medicine, we learn early on in our training to overcome difficulties by simply applying ourselves more diligently, and to deal with challenges by digging in deeper and working all the harder. Without a God who saves, the onus for salvation rests squarely on our shoulders. We are not only responsible to create our own identities, we need to save ourselves, as well. So to meet increasing demands on our practice, we take on more, develop further efficiencies, and lengthen our day, staying late into the evening and coming in on the weekend. Ironically, such a life-style is at odds with care and health. Like old Mother Hubbard going to the cupboard and finding it bare, we too, if left to rely solely upon ourselves, can get spread too thin and burn out with nothing left to give. For many medical practitioners, the heavy workload and associated stresses of self-reliance lead to the development of unhealthy behaviours, including substance abuse and addiction. In a desperate attempt at self-help, some choose to self-medicate. Sadly, medicine is rife with painful examples of once-stellar clinicians who made this error and spiralled downwards into the pit of substance abuse, falling prey to the corrosive effects of addiction.[22] While we often joke about the antioxidant merits of red wine as we mingle at our cocktail parties, we can't afford to forget about the dangers of alcohol and the temptation of drugs. To keep faith in medicine, we need to understand the poverty of self-help approaches, and recognize the risks for both ourselves and our patients.

SUMMARY POINTS – REDEMPTION

1. Our salvation is from God alone

2. The medical cultural narrative of redemption is shaped by self-reliance

3. The false narrative of self-reliance points away from God and leads to unhealthy behaviours

4. Protection from self-reliance can include daily devotional prayer, the spiritual discipline of tithing, and involvement in missional outreach

5. Our role as healthcare providers includes providing our patients with sound teaching and steering them from the divinization of medicine

6. A self-help mindset can lead to a reliance on self-medication and addiction

7. We need to creatively speak words of truth into the lives of our patients who struggle with addiction

8. Ultimate freedom from the bondage of addiction is found in Christ alone

QUESTIONS FOR REFLECTION AND DISCUSSION

1. Have you struggled with self-reliance? How have you addressed this in your life?

2. How would you define tithing? Is this a discipline you have done or see merit in starting?

3. When and where do you best connect with God? Do you have an intentional devotional time in your day?

4. Do you think that God can speak directly into our lives? Have you made use of listening prayer?

5. What are your thoughts about the term, Fear of the Lord? How might you explain this to a new believer?

6. Have you been tempted with Messiah-complex thinking and behaviour? How can we best protect ourselves from this version of self-aggrandizement?

7. Have you struggled with substance addiction or behavioural addiction? How could you use this to help manage a patient's addictive behaviour?

8. What would you say to a fellow believer who confided that they were addicted to pornography? How might you assist them?

CHAPTER NOTES

1. Osler, Sir William. "The Reserves of Life." *St. Mary's Hospital Gazette*, 1907; 13:95-8.

2. Underhill, Evelyn. *The Spiritual Life*. Church Publishing, Inc., 1937.

3. Peterson, Eugene. *Christ Plays in Ten Thousand Places: a conversation in spiritual theology*. Eerdmans, 2005.

4. Nouwen, Henri. *Making All Things New: an invitation to the spiritual life*. Harper One, 1981.

5. *A Guide to Prayer for Ministers and Other Servants*. The Upper Room, 1983.

6. Trueblood, Elton. *The New Man for Our Time*. Harper and Row, 1970.

7. Dickens, Charles. *A Christmas Carol*. Gad's Hill, Higham by Rochester, Kent, 1867.

8. Chambers, Oswald. *My Utmost for His Highest*. Discovery House, 2005.

9. Porter, Roy. *The Greatest Gift to Mankind: A Medical History of Humanity*. W. W. Norton, 1999.

10. Fenton, J.J., Jerant, A.F., Bertakis, K.D., et al. "The Cost of Satisfaction." *Archives of Internal Medicine* 2012; 172:405–11.

11. Boot, J. "Health, Salvation, and the Kingdom of God." *Jubilee* Spring 2012, 11.

12. Moore, J., Fung, J. *The Complete Guide to Fasting: Heal Your Body Through Intermittent, Alternate-Day, and Extended Fasting*. Victory Belt Publishing, 2016.

13. Gordon, E.L., Ariel-Donges, A.H., Bauman, V., Merlo, L. "Nutrients. What Is the Evidence for 'Food Addiction?'" *A Systematic Review*. 2018 Apr; 10(4): 477.

14. O'Campo, P., et al. "Community-Based Services for Homeless Adults Experiencing Concurrent Mental Health and Substance Use Disorders: A Realist Approach to Synthesizing Evidence." *Journal of Urban Health*. November 2009, 86:965.

15. Ng, J. *Canadian Family Physician*. 2017 Nov; 63(11): 866.

16. Leahy, Michael. *Porn Nation: Conquering America's #1 Addiction*. Moody Publishers, 2008.

17. Leahy, *Porn Nation*.

18. Foster, David Kyle. *Sexual Healing Reference Edition: a Biblical Guide to Finding Freedom from Every Major Area of Sexual Sin and Brokenness*. Laurus

Books, 2018.
19. Van Maren, Jonathon. *The Culture War*. Lifecycle Books, 2016.
20. McDowell, Josh. *The Porn Phenomenon: The Impact of Pornography in the Digital Age*. Barna Group ,2016.
21. Foubert, J. *How Pornography Harms: What Today's Teens, Young Adults, Parents, and Pastors need to know*. LifeRich Publishing, 2017.
22. Verghese, A. "Physicians and Addiction." *New England Journal of Medicine*. 2002;346(20):1510–1511.

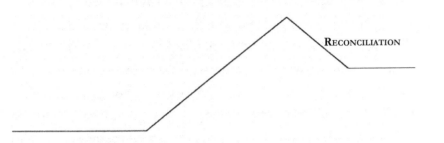

RECONCILIATION

CHAPTER 4

SECULARIZATION AND SELL-OUT

"Whoever wants to be my disciple must deny themselves and take up
their cross and follow me"
Mark 8:43

NO NEUTRAL GROUND

Following the redemptive climax, the denouement segment of the gospel narrative represents our resultant *Reconciliation* with God. Although this feature is placed on the downward segment of the story contour, it's hardly declining in action, particularly for us. Our role here is not a passive one. Rather, this is the participation part of the narrative, where we roll up our sleeves and join with the Holy Spirit, working to bring all things under God's rule and reign. It's a ministry that began at Pentecost, and continues on today to counter the corruption of the world, the flesh, and the Devil, and all that acts to separate us from God's abundant life. With the guidance of the Holy Spirit, our reconciliation efforts are to help right what has gone wrong, straighten what's been twisted, focus what's been distorted, and redirect towards God that which has been pointed aimlessly away.

"Not so," says our culture, which holds to an antithetically different storyline. Steeped in secular humanism, our society promotes the narrative of neutrality, and renders some areas of our lives (the areas that aren't explicitly *religious* in character) as simply non-aligned *common ground*. Neutrality has come to mean an *unbiased position*, and is generally felt to be a good thing. With its veneer of impartiality, it functions as a welcome mat for the modern virtues of inclusivity, tolerance, and diversity. In medicine, the ideas of neutrality are promoted by our use of terms like *reasonable* and *rational* as synonyms for neutrality, and by our demand for *unbiased facts* and a *balanced view* of the issues, as if they were standalone foundational platforms. On the surface, this sort of thinking may seem to ring true; I mean, who wants to be considered biased, right? And besides, some of our activities – like going to church on Sunday and attending a weekly Bible study – are, indeed, God-directed, and other activities – the more regular, day-to-day shopping and goings on – don't seem to point anywhere in particular. However, that's a ruse. It may seem that there's a neutral ground for things, but that's because we live in a humanistic society that promotes a two-realm notion of reality – a religious God-directed realm, and a non-religious *neutered* realm – and because we've been drawn in by the tendrils of secularization and duped.

130

From a biblical worldview, neutrality is a myth, plain and simple. It's a deceptive fabrication that both artificially compartmentalizes our lives intro arbitrary human-constructed divisions, and surreptitiously compromises our faith convictions. As Jeffrey Stout, Professor of Religion at Princeton University once said, "None of us starts from scratch in moral reasoning. We begin already immersed in the assumptions and precedents of a tradition, whether religious or secular."[1] Every thought, word, and deed necessarily either points towards God or points away from Him. There is no middle ground where God doesn't lay claim, and not one square inch that's been left undisputed between Jesus and Satan. It's an all or none universe. Hudson Taylor, the famed Christian missionary to China summarized it well by saying, "if not Lord of all, then not Lord at all." We need to appreciate that facts aren't solitary entities that can float around independently. Every fact must be anchored in relationship to other facts in order to be comprehensible. And to be meaningful, all facts must ultimately be in relationship to the absolute, personal God of Scripture, who governs all things and gives them meaning. The Father of Lies uses the myth of neutrality to his advantage, first by compartmentalizing our lives into the sacred and the secular, and then by expanding the secular parts to involve most things.

The consequence of buying into this clever illusion is that it redirects our energies away from God. Instead of seeing ourselves as invited into the ministry of reconciliation as co-laborers with the Holy Spirit, we slowly begin to see ourselves on the rat race of eking out a living. As this takes place, our efforts can easily get reduced from an intended priestly calling to a mere secular enterprise. If left unchecked, our values and ethics soon follow suit and become shaped more by public opinion than by holy Scripture. Unless we take intentional steps to protect ourselves from secularization, we run the risk of becoming no different than non-Christians in thought, word and deed. If this becomes the case, then the critical areas of our lives that once separated us from the world, the flesh, and the devil, will do so no longer and we'll lose our saltiness. And then, when important issues arise in the public sphere, which attack Christian foundations and necessitate a defense, our go-to response may simply be one of complacency and compromise.

SANCTIFICATION NOT SECULARIZATION

Although I had grown up in the church and was raised and nurtured in biblical thought, I didn't always talk that way or walk it, particularly in medical school. Far from it. At that time, my interests were geared more towards partying than praising. It's not that I saw my med school days as one big party; it was more that I saw them as a series of big parties all joined together by intense studying. Embarrassingly, I was no exception to the adage that *preacher's kids are the worst*, and happily joined in with the shenanigans and debauchery along with everyone else. Well, almost everyone. There were a few visible Christians in our medical school class who didn't partake in our tomfoolery – the *Holy Joes*, as we called them. One fellow student stands out in particular for me. I knew that he was a Christian right from the get-go by the cross he wore around his neck, and by the fact that he listed teaching Sunday school on the class brief-bio page. As part of a Christian club on campus, he would often stand up during class announcements, and tell us about various upcoming events, even taking some flak from our class feminists when he mentioned the Pro-life Rally. Some of my peers called him "Father Mulcahey" from M.A.S.H. because one of them had seen him praying with a patient on the ward.

I didn't have much involvement with him until our clinical rotations overlapped at the Women's Pavilion. I overheard him inform his surgical mentor at the beginning of the surgical slate that he wouldn't be taking part in any abortions during his gynecology rotation. I caught this because I happened to be in the very operating room he was exiting, and was already involved in the very case he was washing his hands of. I was surprised by his courage, and felt embarrassed that the thought of not participating in abortions hadn't crossed my mind. At that time, however, I was more concerned about getting medical experiences than considering their ethical nature. So, disguised behind my surgical mask, I dutifully carried on with my involvement with the case, as well as with the two dozen additional abortion cases that followed that day.

Later, when I saw him waiting at the bus stop, I made some polite conversation and asked him if he was planning to join in the competition against the other medical student years and attend the annual Great Gurney Race. His answer also surprised me; not that he declined from our fun run, but that he said "no" because he wanted to "keep the Sabbath." I knew full well that he meant "go to church," but I'd never heard anyone refer to it in that way before, and certainly would never have considered swapping a morning's amusement for some boring church service myself. Church pews and piety were for the dead and dying, I thought. I wanted to embrace life and all the fun that could be had in doing so. But to keep the conversation going, I asked him what church he attended, and mentioned in passing that I also went to church (purposely neglecting to mention how infrequently I attended). Then he took me off guard once more by saying, "Really? You're a Christian? I wouldn't have known that about you."

I was speechless. And although his quizzical response hurt me to the core, it shouldn't have. How could he possibly have known that I was a baptized believer? In honest reflection, I wasn't living a Christian life in any shape or form. My role as a medical student on campus didn't extend beyond the narrow reaches of the library, swimming pool, and pub. In the public sphere, I was completely disconnected and largely unaware of the issues pressing in on Christian ethics and the global church. And in my personal circle, I was no different than my friends, partying like the rest of them, uninvolved in Bible study or Christian outreach, and attending church only sporadically, and then only reluctantly. Although my baptism vows had been sincere at the time, and I believed that I'd been washed and sanctified, I wasn't living my life set apart. I'd allowed myself to fall in step with secular society, rather than keeping in step with the Holy Spirit. I had become a secular humanist, a wolf in sheep's clothing.

SABBATH AS A SHIELD FROM SECULARIZATION

Since we are immersed in the secular world of medicine, we need to protect ourselves from having our lives compartmentalized into the secular and sacred, and from having our work reduced to a worldly undertaking. Sabbath-keeping is central to this task. As a spiritual discipline, keeping the Sabbath keeps us in step with the Holy Spirit and, in the words of Eugene Peterson, "sets an important rhythm to our lives."[2] With its biblical context found in the Genesis week of creation, Sabbath is connected to God's ongoing covenantal relationship with creation and serves as a point of transition between God's creative work and His providential governing of all things. The Torah ordinance – to keep the Sabbath holy – sets a clear demarcation between labour and rest, and in so doing, promotes human flourishing by directing us to operate within our design specifications. Famed British psychiatrist, Sir James Crichton-Browne, who was well-acquainted with our physical need for rest, once said, "We doctors, in the treatment of nervous disease, are now constantly compelled to prescribe periods of rest. Some periods are, I think, only Sundays in arrears." By establishing the work/rest cycle, Sabbath keeping helps align us with God's creational rhythm, and fosters the blessings of life, including the health of our body and the nurture of our soul.

Prioritizing the Sabbath in our week prioritizes God in our lives, and making it a day of rest helps protect us from the idolatry of work. Unfortunately, in the 24/7 world of healthcare provision, this isn't always possible. The realities of shift work, hospital-coverage schedules, and on-call rotas unavoidably interfere with even the most diligent Sabbath-keeping rhythm. However, occasionally breaking this rhythm in order to fulfill our healthcare duties doesn't mean we'll lose sight of God in our lives. As important as the Sabbath is for protecting us from secularization, keeping it was not intended as an end in itself either. As Jesus emphasized, "The Sabbath was made for man, not man for the Sabbath" (Mark 2:27). This is one area that the Pharisees got wrong. In biblical times, religious authorities had given Sabbath keeping a life of its own, mandating hundreds of rules around the day of rest, and making it more of a burden than a blessing. These legalistic interpretations of Sabbath keeping were of central concern to Jesus – the Lord of the Sabbath – and led to numerous confrontations with the Pharisees. My Sabbath-keeping exceptions are my loss, and only prove to me the importance of the rule. As Abraham Lincoln said, "As we keep or break the Sabbath day, we nobly save or meanly lose the last best hope by which man rises." On the occasions when I've had to work on Sunday and can't make it to church with my family, I've usually tried to find some other way to mark the day holy. Sometimes I take in an early-morning downtown communion service before starting my hospital rounds, or occasionally, I've sat in on portions of the ecumenical service held in our hospital chapel after rounds. If my work responsibilities even prevent this, then I block off some time in the week for journaling and biblical reflection. Intentionally setting aside time in my workweek this way is like making an appointment with the Lord. It helps remind me that

God is sovereign over every part of my life, and underscore that my times are in His hands (Ps. 31:14-5).

In our present era, the issue with Sabbath keeping is less about getting time off work, and more about how we choose to fill that time. We live in an age of unprecedented amounts of leisure time in which there are a vast array of activities that contend for our attention. Everybody's working for the weekend, it seems. However, that work can be misdirected if the leisure time we're gunning towards points us away from God. The Sabbath was made for man, to be sure, but not so we can recover from Saturday night's debauchery, or bask in self-indulgent me-time. Nor was the Sabbath made so we can catch up on paperwork, or tackle projects from the towering to-do lists. This sort of utilitarian break merely exchanges one type of work for another. And in this case, a change is *not* just as good as a rest. Although the word, Sabbath, literally means quit or rest, the quitting and resting isn't simply from labour. Just as a Sunday spent as a hedonistic holiday is a misuse of the Sabbath, so too is frantically catching up on household chores or shopping till we're dropping. There was good reason why stores were mandated closed on Sundays in days past. Having stores operating at full capacity on Sundays has plunged our society into a seven-day work week enslavement, promoting ever more unabashedly the idolatry of materialism. The Pharisees with their legalistic rules around Sabbath may have been in error, but we now face the opposite error in this permissive disregard for God's Fourth Commandment in His Law. So, while we need to be good stewards of time, we should never consider Sabbath keeping a waste of time.

Sabbath keeping allows us to formally enter into God's presence and get to know His voice. There are so many distractions that bombard us during the work week and so few opportunities to turn them off. Sabbath keeping is just such a time when we can turn off the noise of life. As Oswald Chambers said, "The busyness of things obscures our concentration on God … Never let a hurried lifestyle disturb the relationship of abiding in Him. This is an easy thing to allow, but we must guard against it."[3] When we keep the Sabbath, we guard ourselves by quieting the monkey in our mind, and offering our undivided attention to our Maker. Resting in Him in quiet meditation and prayer can allow us to feel the nudging of the Holy Spirit and better discern the godly direction for our lives. This protects us from either neglecting to follow His call for our lives – choosing a handy lifestyle over a life styled by His hand – or to misinterpret His call and misdirect our energies. This is important to be aware of since we've also been given the warning: "Not everyone who says to me, 'Lord, Lord,' will enter the kingdom of heaven, but only the one who does the will of my Father who is in heaven" (Matt. 7:21). God-inspired work needs to begin by first resting in Him and hearing His bidding for our lives. It follows then, that Sunday should be considered the first day of our week, when we do this sort of resting, and not the last day of the week, when we do everything but. Although the Sabbath was the seventh and final day of Creation in which "God rested from all His work which He had done" (Gen. 2:2), it marked Adam's first day. So, just as God rested and was fully present to man on the first Sabbath, we, too, are to rest and be fully present to Him as we mark the present Sabbath.

Sabbath keeping is not a solitary enterprise, either. To participate fully in the Sabbath, we need to be an active part of a holy community. The challenge, of course, is finding a biblically-focussed community of faith amongst the many social justice groups, nominal congregations, and social club churches. Secularization has not only taken hold of our society, it's invaded the church as well, diluting and distorting the life-saving message of salvation. Many churches today seem to offer their parishioners a watered-down version of the gospel, with little more than pop-psychology support and direction. Carlo Carretto candidly expressed this frustration by lamenting, "How baffling you are, oh Church, and yet how I love you! ... I have seen nothing in the world more devoted to obscurity, more compromised, more false, and I have touched nothing more pure, more generous, more beautiful. How often I have wanted to shut the doors of my soul in your face, and how often I have prayed to die in the safety of your arms... and where should I go?"[4] Sadly, such churches seem more concerned with being considered *relevant* and keeping their tax-exemption charitable status, than holding to sound doctrine or proclaiming biblical truth. Ironically, these very churches seem to struggle the most with dwindling membership. And perhaps this is best, since as Greg Bahnsen said, "When the church begins to look and sound like the world, there is no compelling rationale for its continued existence."[5]

As vexing as the secularization of the church seems, it doesn't represent the demise of Christianity, but is rather a refining process for the body of Christ. While nominal churches diminish and close, biblically focussed communities of faith are continuing to grow and prosper. As the anti-Christian sentiments of our culture become more hostile, it may come to pass that the visible church follows the path of the European cathedrals and, as institution, gets reduced to historical relic. But as the growing Chinese Christian church bears bold witness, persecution only strengthens the body of believers. The church as organization might shrink and die, but the church as *organism* is still alive and well. Pentecost gave birth to the church as a believing body of Christ's disciples and Sabbath keeping as a celebration of Christ's victory over death. As such, the Sabbath preceded the church institution, and our faithful Sabbath keeping needs to continue in spite of whatever local waywardness.

THE PROTECTION OF PRAISE AND THANKSGIVING

Establishing a Sabbath rhythm to the week can go a long way to stave off the creep of secularization in our lives, but it may not be enough to safeguard us from the lure of compartmentalization and complacency. Our minds need to be daily protected from every secular thought, particularly within the material workplace of healthcare provision. Incorporating regular praise and adopting a mind frame of thanksgiving can help afford us such protection. Having praise and thanksgiving on our lips best aligns our lives in God-honoring service, and helps to protect us from the artificial separation of our lives into the secular and sacred realms. As the apostle Paul commands, "Rejoice in the Lord always… with thanksgiving… and the peace of God which transcends all understanding will guard your hearts and your minds in Christ Jesus" (Phil. 4:4-7). By starting each day with praise, we set a fresh God-directed tone for our work ahead. And by incorporating moments of thanksgiving throughout our day, we keep ourselves ever mindful of God's manifold mercies and abundant blessings.

The important link between daily praise and healthcare provision became evident to me while I was on mission in Cameroon. Working at the Mbingo Baptist Church Hospital, I joined the other hospital staff in their daily Chapel-time. With the first light of dawn every morning, the pews of the sizeable sanctuary would be filled to capacity with nurses, pharmacists, social workers, orderlies, lab technicians, custodial staff, physicians and surgeons. At 6:30am sharp, the djembe drums would begin beating and the singing would break out, accompanied by swaying movements and raised arms. While there was also a brief homily delivered by one of the hospital chaplains, it was the music that moved me. With the songs of praise playing over in my mind, I found myself excited to see patients and take an active role in God's ministry of reconciliation in medicine. When I returned home, I continued the discipline of morning praise, minus the drums and hand waving. Since I couldn't lay my hands on any authentic African gospel-styled music, I resorted to listening to various Western praise selections. Although they pale by comparison to the African rhythms and harmonies, my chorus selections provide a platform of praise nonetheless, and underscore the reality that "God inhabits the praises of his people" (Ps. 22:3 KJV).

The imperative to be thankful rings throughout the old and new testaments of Scripture, and for good reason. By incorporating praise and thanksgiving into the bustle of our everyday tasks and work week we can better keep focussed on God and his providential care for us. The apostle Paul sets the bar particularly high when he says, "Rejoice always, pray continually, give thanks in all circumstances; for this is God's will for you in Christ Jesus" (1 Thes. 5:16-18). It's quite a gauntlet, and easier said than done, especially on those bad days when everything that could go wrong seems to. However, Paul didn't restrict his thanksgiving to only *good days*; and reading his graphic account with the experiences of hunger and thirst, several floggings, and numerous shipwrecks, he had quite the number of *bad days*, and far worse than any day I've yet experienced (2 Cor. 11). So, this recurring imperative to be thankful is likely in part because appreciation and thankfulness don't come naturally. Our fallen nature is one of self-entitlement, self-reliance, and taking things for granted. God commands us in the Bible to adopt praise and thanksgiving in order to rescue us from ourselves.

Fortunately for me, He's also given me numerous formative role models of a grateful heart. My uncle Edmund was a formative example of someone who modeled this essential behaviour. He was a German pastor who lived through both wars, the First as a refugee from Russia and the Second as a prisoner in a Russian POW camp. Despite the horrors he endured, he maintained a deep sense of gratitude, which permeated every aspect of his life. In fact, he reminded me of the little old man from Robert Redford's film, *The Milagro Bean Field War*. Similar to that character, the first words out of his mouth on rising in the morning were, "Gott sei Dank!" or "Let God be thanked." As a young boy, I found it puzzling that whenever I would thank him for something, like the lunch meal, or a treat or toy, he would consistently reply with the same emphatic phrase, "Gott sei Dank, Gott sei Dank!" When I asked my dad about why Uncle always directed everything back to God, he told me that the war had been hard on him.

"Oh, you mean he got hurt and now isn't right in the head?" I asked, thinking that brain injury might also explain some of his other more age-related idiosyncrasies.

"No," my Dad replied with a patient smile, "I mean, he experienced some pretty horrible things in Russia during the war, and knows what the world looks like when God is excluded… and that every good thing is a gift from God. He's reminding us in his own way, you see, that we should be thankful to God for all things and all the time."

Nobel Peace Prize laureate, Albert Schweitzer was another example of someone who demonstrated a gratitude-informed life. Masterfully combining the talents of music, preaching, writing, medicine, and surgery, he was an early inspiration for me. As an accomplished organist and renowned expert on Bach, he would go on European concert tours to fund his mission hospital in Lambaréné, Gabon. Schweitzer's fundamental guiding principle was one of gratitude in all things, and he would say, "He who does not reflect his life back to God in gratitude does not know himself."[6] While I disagreed with his pantheistic spirituality, I continue to regard him as an important role model for effectively incorporating the Christian faith into his medical practice, and for his unwavering emphasis on thanksgiving to God.

Growing up as a family, we expressed our thankfulness on a regular basis by folding our hands, bowing our heads, and 'saying Grace' before each meal, usually offered by my father. However, the apostle Paul encourages us to push our God-directed expressions of gratitude further, beyond the confines of the mealtime, and "give thanks in all circumstances" (1 Thes. 5:17). This implies that we not only give thanks frequently throughout the day, meal or no meal, but we do so regardless of whether our present situation is a favorable one or not – in sickness or in health, for better or for worse. This is a tall order and, like a marriage vow, goes against the grain of our self-focussed quick-to-complain nature. But in order to break the white-knuckle grip of secularization on our lives, it's important that we develop a deep sense of godly gratitude that is impervious to our momentary circumstances. In order to do so, we need to remember why it is that we're thankful in the first place – that God created us in His image, that He has promised not to abandon us in our sufferings, that He died to rescue us and is our source of salvation, that He co-labours with us in our work, and that He has included us in His eternal plans – and keep this gospel truth fixed in the forefront of our minds at all times and in all circumstances. In this way, regardless of how our day begins or transpires, we can be sincerely grateful. It works in the opposite direction as well; by intentionally incorporating moments of thanksgiving sprinkled throughout our day – from praise for the dawn of a new morning to thanksgiving for a safe arrival home at day's end – we keep ourselves mindful of God's mercies and blessings. In this way, we are more likely to live out our faith in medicine as a priestly calling.

THE JESUS WAY

As the spiritual discipline of Sabbath keeping becomes established in our lives and extended into our work week by the daily activities of praise and thanksgiving, the cosmic battle between the Kingdom of

God and the kingdoms of the world becomes all the more evident, and the need for the ministry of reconciliation all the more urgent. Once the illusion of neutrality has been dispelled and the division of our lives into the artificial realms of sacred and secular dismantled, it's easier to appreciate the distinction between what is God-honoring and what is not. "Those who call evil good and good evil, who put darkness for light and light for darkness, who put bitter for sweet and sweet for bitter" (Is. 5:20), stand out like red flags. So it's no longer a question of whether or not there's a role for reconciliation, or if we should involve ourselves or not; we are called to "demolish arguments and every pretension that sets itself up against the knowledge of God" (2 Cor. 10:5). The questions at hand are *where* do we start, and *how* do we best go about this ministry of reconciliation.

In terms of *where* we should start, the answer, simply enough, is where we're presently standing. God has placed us where we are for good reason. Since the Holy Spirit indwells us, in a very real sense, where we are standing at any given moment in time is holy ground, and represents our mission field. Within the reach of this stance is our professional sphere of healthcare provision, our personal sphere of friends, colleagues, and fellow church parishioners, and the public sphere of politics and social media. Although the biblical foundation for engaging each of these spheres will be similar, our approach, choice of words, and our emphasis will differ depending on the context. In our professional sphere with patients, for example, our primary role will be one of advocacy and healthcare educator. Using welcoming language of encouragement, our emphasis in the clinical setting will be to provide comprehensive medical care with attention on the whole-person needs of our patients. In our personal circle with family and close friends, however, our role will be more pastoral and one of support, encourage-ment, and accountability. In those intimate settings, our approach will be less formal with more listening than counsel. Using winsome and tender language, our emphasis will be to foster trusting communication and deepen relationships. In the public sphere, by contrast, our role will be one of social conscience and will require courage. But as is emphasized in Scripture, "If you do not stand firm in your faith, you will not stand at all" (Is. 7:9). Here, as we exercise our civic responsibility in addressing the hot-button issues of our day, our approach will require a defensive tack. In order to re-establish Christian values in our society, our emphasis will need to be more strategic, and our language carefully chosen.

In terms of the *how-to* part of our reconciling ministry, it's important that we remain biblically faithful and ensure that our methods fit with our message. As the apostle Paul reminds us, "For though we live in the world, we do not wage war as the world does. The weapons we fight with are not the weapons of the world" (2 Cor. 10:3-4). This necessitates, regardless of how our opposition may choose to operate, that we restrict ourselves to the high road. William Ralph Inge observed that "The enemies of freedom do not argue; they shout and they shoot."[7] Our means to advance the Kingdom of God can't be accomplished with hostile protests, petty argumentation, slander, or ad hominem smear campaigns. Eugene Peterson makes this point by emphasizing that "Ways and means that are removed or abstracted from Jesus and the Scriptures that give witness to him amount sooner or later to a betrayal of Jesus."[8] It follows then that the ways and means we adopt should be in keeping with and reflect Jesus' ministry. He is the *Great Physician* after all, and our best role model for all reconciling engagements. Although the question, "*What Would Jesus Do?*" may seem trite and smack of bumper-sticker spirituality, I think that a *WWJD* approach is worth considering to check and balance our efforts.

Central and unique to the ministry of Jesus was His balance of grace and truth. This was emphasized in the prologue to John's Gospel, "For the law was given through Moses; grace and truth came through Jesus Christ" (John 1:16-17). Calling the religious leaders to task, Jesus held fast to biblical truth, and underscored that "not the smallest letter, not the least stroke of a pen, will by any means disappear from the Law" (Matt. 5:18). And while He maintained this unwavering commitment to the letter of the Law, He simultaneously welcomed sinners and outcasts with an unlimited offer of grace, saying "Come to me, all you who are weary and burdened, and I will give you rest" (Matt. 11:28). When the woman caught in adultery was brought before Jesus, He didn't legalistically dismiss her with disdain and disgust, allowing the rocks to fly; nor did He neglect the biblical sexual ethic by affirming her sexual behaviour and celebrating her promiscuous lifestyle. Rather, He said, "Go and sin no more" (John 8:11) and, standing between the armed mob and the accused, He protected her from harm and offered her abundant life free from the slavery of sin. Not easy to do, but certainly food for thought as we consider the *how-to* aspects of reconciliation.

The Jesus way is not one of condemnation, nor is it one of unconditional acceptance and approval. God loves us as we are, to be sure; but He doesn't want to leave us in our sorry state of self-saturated sin. God is holy. And since He created us to be in relationship with Him, He wants us to be holy, as well. As George MacDonald said, "The Lord never came to deliver men from the consequences of their sins while yet those sins remained: that would be to cast out of the window the medicine of cure while yet the man lay sick."[9] Rather, God desires our transformation, so that grace and truth can abide in our lives, and we can be ambassadors of Christ and messengers of reconciliation. While grace balanced with truth produces an unavoidable degree of tension, analogous to a crossbow, for example, it's a tension that's necessary to function. The bow is only effective when under the pull of the bowstring on each stave. Without the string being held taut, the crossbow is useless and becomes little more than an unusually bent stick – not even suitable for walking on flat ground. Likewise, we need to maintain this kind of tension between grace and truth. Failing to maintain the pull between Christ's exclusive claim to the truth and His inclusive compassion, we render our reconciling efforts futile. If we capitulate on biblical truth, we forfeit the gospel and its redeeming power; yet if we fail to reach out in compassion and care, we miss the opportunity to witness and share the gospel. Despite the best of our intentions, we become "like a bow gone slack" (Hos. 7:16 REV) and will altogether miss the most critical mark.

Putting Servanthood into Practice

Jesus repeatedly demonstrated for His disciples how the tension of grace and truth is to be worked out in the day-to-day fray. He didn't just use words though; His actions also spoke volumes. To provide them with an indelible image of Kingdom-directed leadership, and "show them the full extent of His love" (John 13:1), He took on a servant's role, and on the night He was betrayed, washed His disciples' feet. This gospel account of servanthood was poignantly illustrated to me when I happened upon a foot washing ceremony at a local German evangelical church. In the hopes of improving my faltering second language, I attended an evening mid-week prayer service. I was following along pretty well until halfway through when we were instructed to stand. With my limited comprehension, I was confused why the congregation suddenly divided down gender lines, with the women walking into one adjoining room, and we men marched downstairs. I remained confused until I saw a series of water basins and towels set up on the tables. Then it dawned on me that Easter was fast approaching, and figured that foot washing was probably one of the ways they marked the Passion Week. Sure enough, we all paired up and everyone started removing their footwear. I was a bit self-conscious removing my odorous Oxfords. It had been a long day, and I had come straight from the hospital to the service, with no time to freshen up. So, when I peeled off my sweaty dress socks, and placed my feet into the water-filled basin, I felt some embarrassment when sock lint and debris floated to the surface. However, once the foot washing began, my awkwardness with the situation vanished along with the toe jam. Language barrier aside, I was taken aback by the profound nature of the ceremony. The intimacy of the foot washing exchange produced an immediate kindred bond between myself and the gentleman I was paired with. The combination of performing the menial task and receiving personal care produced feelings of humility and vulnerability, simultaneously. The whole experience gave me a deeper appreciation for the central role of servanthood in Christian life and its important example for reconciling witness. I often reflect upon this during my regular night-time routine. As I perch myself on our narrow bathroom counter and fill the sink with water as hot as I can take to wash the lint out from between my own toes, I think about Jesus humbly washing those twelve pairs of dirty feet, and the call on my own life to be a servant to others.

Applied to the practice of medicine, an attitude of servanthood can set the stage for the provision of empathetic care and the witness of Christ's inclusive compassion. Acts of servanthood can push us out of our comfort zones and expose the more vulnerable and tender aspects of our characters. The humble provision of personal care for our patients can pull us off the high horse of indifference, and allow us to interact with them on a more intimate level. At such times, we are more likely to appreciate our patients as "fellow travellers to the grave and not another race of creatures bound on other journeys,"[10] and we are in a better position to see them the way God sees them – as his dearly beloved children. Servanthood makes tangible the words of Jesus when He said, "Whatever you do for one of the least of these, you do for me" (Matt. 25:40). In a very real sense, when we reach out to our patients with the attitude of a servant, we become the hands and feet of Jesus. With this in mind, even menial tasks take on new depth of meaning. Understanding the holy in the humble, we no longer begrudge having to chase the missing lab results with repeated phone calls or filling out the patient's multi-paged insurance form. A servant mindset allows us to better endure the incessant overhead pages and brutal wake-up calls, and to transcend the stench of the commode and the obscenities yelled in delirium down the hall.

An attitude of servanthood allows us to provide our undivided attention to patient care amid hectic work schedules, and to look for opportunities to speak words of truth and life into their lives. Considered this way, all of our everyday clinical interactions take on new depth and timely opportunity. When we spot a patient struggling in identity crisis, for example, a servant mindset can goad us to foster a safe and trusting relationship by communicating in word and deed their significance and acceptance. Likewise, an attitude of servanthood can spur us to come alongside our suffering patients with not only analgesics, but with a creative approach to bring meaning into their distress and despair. The humble posturing of servanthood also allows us to counter the divinization of medicine, and puts us into a better position to direct patients away from potential destructive ends and towards life-giving solutions instead. By having an ear attuned to the Holy Spirit, servanthood opens up the opportunities to gently witness and share the gospel with those who hunger for its message.

As our modus operandi in the clinical setting, servanthood can allow us to balance the tension between grace and truth, and provide us the means to bring reconciliation into the sphere of medicine. This is the case because it's God whom we are serving, not primarily our patients, and certainly not ourselves. Servanthood allows us to balance care and compassion with biblical truth because it directs our efforts heavenward. Our priestly role in medicine is not a self-service exercise to pat our egos and pad our pockets; nor is it a rash response to carry out our patients' every wish and whim. We are not the centerpiece of our calling, nor are our patients; that place is reserved for God alone. Jesus grounded His servanthood in knowing where He was coming from and where He was going. As the gospel recounts, "Jesus knew that the Father had put all things under his power, and that he had come from God and was returning to God; so he got up from the meal, took off his outer clothing, and wrapped a towel around his waist... and began to wash his disciples' feet" (John 13:3-5). Likewise, in order to live out our faith in medicine, we need to know where we are coming from and where we are going. Both what we do and where we direct what we do are critically important. Only when we have our identity in Christ firmly established and our medical work intentionally God-directed, can we effectively work alongside the Holy Spirit to bring about reconciliation into the secularized sphere of medicine.

CHRIST IN CONFLICT

Servanthood not only presses us to provide compassionate care, its humble posture points that care away from ourselves and towards God. Analogous to an arrow of a mathematical vector, which has both content and direction, our medical work also has body and bearing. It's important to keep this in mind, since, although we may go all out for our patients – getting that second blanket from the warmer or helping them to the commode – we must never go in a direction that leads us away from God or is counter to His revealed truth. The substance of our medical care must always remain Christ centered. And here's the rub: what do we do when the will of our patient clashes with our understanding of God's will? At certain unavoidable times, we may be faced with a patient who requests some pill or procedure that goes contrary to our biblically informed conscience. This is to be expected and even anticipated. We can't expect our non-believing patients to make their decisions and live their lives in accordance with the Bible. Nonetheless, we must endeavor to do so, and at all times, and in all places. During these times of potential conflict, it may be tempting to let our bow of grace and truth go slack a bit on the truth part, and simply comply with our patient's request. We can always parrot the popular refrain, "It's their body" and hide behind the rationalization that "we're merely providing a service." However, by surrendering the biblical truth claims on our lives, we end up forfeiting the gospel and its redeeming power, both for our salvation and our patients' welfare. Even though a non-confrontational path may be a popular way of practicing medicine and seem easier, it's not the Jesus way. Jesus may have been meek and mild in certain contexts, but he was no pushover. When confronted with the money-changers in the temple, for example, who had turned the house of prayer into a "den of thieves" (Matt. 21:13), "he made a whip out of cords, and drove all from the temple area," scattering coins and overturning tables in the process, all out of zeal for His Father's house (John 2:15-17). Even when faced with the grim spectre of the fateful cup of wrath, Jesus didn't shirk his responsibility to the truth, but obediently said to the Father, "yet not my will, but yours be done" (Luke 22:42).

So, if we truly care for our patients, and actually want them to flourish, we may have to disagree with some of their lifestyle and health choices. To maintain our commitment to biblical truth, we may have to say 'no' to patient requests or at least decline our involvement. In preparation for God-directed servanthood in healthcare, it's worthwhile anticipating certain potential conflict circumstances, and consider beforehand how we might best navigate with grace and truth our patient involvement. What follows are three such scenarios for reflection.

A CASE OF GENDER REASSIGNMENT

The first scenario is one of a patient who has rejected God's design of their body and expresses a desire to undergo gender reassignment surgery. How might we demonstrate our compassion for someone struggling with a sexuality-based identity like this, while at the same time maintain our allegiance to biblical truth? And is it even possible? Of course, contemporary policy makers would say that it isn't, and to simply shelf the Bible and make the patient's plea our priority. Reminiscent of George Orwell's allegorical dystopia, *Animal Farm*, "Four Legs Good, Two Legs Better," they hold to the view that the rights of some – the patient – supersede those of others – the healthcare professional.

While it may not be possible to both satisfy the patient and maintain our biblical integrity, it's a worthy goal to attempt. The starting point is fostering a trusting relationship with the patient. We need to provide them a welcoming clinical environment, and apply our best medical skills to reduce their healthcare discrepancies and ensure they're properly cared for. Next, it's important for us to engender a broader definition of their identity by communicating that we accept them as they are – beyond their gender designation or sexual preferences – and that they have significance in our eyes. Then, within the context of our caregiver/patient relationship, we can share some of our concerns about their surgical request, outlining the limited and often short-lived benefits, the irreversible harm, and the patient regret that commonly follows such a decision.[11] Recognizing that the surgically fabricated and hormonally-induced transgender world fails to address the underlying deep-seated psychological issues, we can emphasize these medical misgivings without having to directly reference the Bible. Out of these clinical concerns, we can encourage them to choose a less invasive and irreversible option to address their symptoms of dysphoria, or at least to allow some time to pass before proceeding. Of course, there are ethical issues to bear in mind with these less invasive interventions as well. Medications used to block puberty with cross-sex hormones of testosterone or estrogen can have irreversible effects in children, and have been associated with numerous health risks, including vascular disease and cancer.[12] However, if we insist on a hard line without any room for compromise, we may jeopardize our relationship with the patient, and put ourselves at risk for not only professional rebuke, but public censure. Besides, studies have shown that patients in these positions often do change their minds on their own accord and decide to forgo surgical reassignment.[13] Nevertheless, if despite our best relational efforts, they demand to proceed with their original request for surgery, our biblically faithful response is to decline involvement. We need to be honest and communicate that while we appreciate their struggle, we can't support their decision as a solution that is in their best interest. We can still try to maintain our hard-earned relationship with them and continue to be involved in their general care, but we cannot condone or facilitate this kind of decision that points away from God.

A CASE OF ABORTION REQUEST

The second scenario for consideration is that of a young woman requesting an abortion. Our culture has done its best to either dismiss abortion as a non-issue, or to utilize intimidating slogans of rights and freedoms as a smokescreen to hide its horror. However, despite the widespread complacency or rhetorical terrorism and camouflage, the killing of the preborn is not compatible with Christian healthcare practice. As the Psalmist laments, "They shed innocent blood, the blood of their sons and daughters... and the land was desecrated" (Ps. 106:37-38). So, with this biblical prohibition in mind, how then might we provide compassionate care for a woman carrying an unwanted pregnancy, while at the same time defending the sanctity of her baby's life? Although this is a hyper-polarized, emotionally supercharged topic, the clinical starting point is not one of argument. Our role is to first come alongside the patient and listen rather than to speak. It's important to recognize from the outset that such a decision on the part of an expectant mother is commonly fraught with inner turmoil, and often represents a desperate measure for desperate times. So, rather than either automatically agreeing to make termination arrangements, or flatly refusing to take any part in the deed, we need to do our utmost to first engage the patient relationally, and understand the impetus behind the request. Is the pregnancy unwanted because of youth, school demands or career pressures? Or is the decision to terminate the pregnancy due to the lack of emotional supports or financial resources? Perhaps the patient is being pressured by a boyfriend or family member, or perhaps the baby is disabled in some way or was the product of sexual assault. Knowing this answer can help us better empathize with the patient's struggles, and frame the alternative life-giving options that are available. As well, understanding the backstory to their request can allow us to better unpack the truth that aborting the baby does nothing to solve the problems at hand, but in fact, only compounds them. School and career pressures press on, financial strains continue to loom, relational tensions persist, and abuse recovery limps forward. Abortion only adds to the misery.

The request for an abortion is an opportunity for us to underscore the preciousness of human life. This reality can be made real with the aid of a fetal heart monitor, or poignantly illustrated with abdominal ultrasound imaging. Similar to the epiphany dramatized in the film *Unplanned*, if the realness of the unborn baby can be revealed, the idea of termination becomes all the more unthinkable. If we don't have the time to provide this level of counselling, we should refer patients on to pro-life organizations that do.[14] Across the street from the abortion clinic at my hospital, for example, is a pregnancy resource center that offers information to women about their pregnancy options, including adoption and parenting, and offers pre- and post-abortion counseling, as well as birthing assistance.[15] They have trained personnel on hand who can listen, offer valuable perspective, and provide needed support to expectant mothers contemplating abortion. There's an urgency here; lives are in the balance. As Christian healthcare providers, we cannot faithfully condone or facilitate the act of abortion, which directly violates Holy Scripture. There is no middle ground here. Our legal conscience rights in Canada might currently be in a compromised position, but our witness on this life-threatening issue can't afford to be. If, despite our best efforts to listen, advise, and provide referral for life-affirming help, the patient still demands to proceed with ending her baby's life, our response must be to decline our involvement. We can hope for an ongoing relationship with the patient, but we can't condone or facilitate killing.

A CASE OF ASSISTED SUICIDE REQUEST

This third scenario for consideration is that of a patient requesting euthanasia. Similar to abortion, *medical assistance in dying* (MAID) – or to use the more accurate and less euphemistic term, *assisted suicide* – also opposes the foundational biblical view of the sanctity of human life. As Moses warned, "Whoever sheds human blood, by humans shall their blood be shed; for in the image of God has God made mankind" (Gen. 9:6). With this caution in mind, we need to consider how we can provide compassionate care for someone asking to die, yet at the same time defend the sanctity of the very life they are desiring to discard. While contemporary medical and legal authorities may presently demand from healthcare practitioners either direct involvement in the MAID process or, at the very least, complicit involvement with the provision of a referral, it needs to be emphasized that any involvement in the taking of an innocent life, including euthanasia, is antagonistic to the traditions of medical care as practiced from antiquity, and is diametrically opposed to Christian healthcare provision. So, regardless of whatever the legal repercussions may be, we cannot in good conscience facilitate the practice of euthanasia in any way.

Similar to the abortion case, if the request for assisted suicide arises within the context of the patient/practitioner relationship, our response is not to be one of argument. We need to appreciate from the outset that the desire for assisted suicide is a symptom of an unmet need. So, rather than countering with an antagonistic apologetic, a far more effective and fruitful approach in this context is ask them questions as to the *why* of their wish. In order to determine the basis for their expressed suffering, it's important that we take the time to listen to their story and struggles. Analogous to a patient presenting with shortness of breath, our task is to uncover the etiology of the dyspnea. Like Dorothy's terrier, Toto, from The Wizard of Oz, we need to look behind the curtain and get to the root cause of their struggles and uncover what's driving their death desire. Is their request to die stemming from a loss of bodily control or the feeling of helplessness? Is it the fear of futility or the fear of the unknown? Are they lonely or feel abandoned? Are they requesting death because they feel they are a burden on their family or on society? By understanding the underlying issues, we can better come alongside them in their suffering, and creatively look for ways to bring meaning into their distress.

Since the request for euthanasia is essentially a cry for help, it's important that we respond by reminding them of their inherent value and their fuller identity beyond their illness. If, however, despite our best relational efforts and creative suggestions, they remain resolute on choosing death, our response must be to decline our involvement. We can walk with them through the valley of the shadow of death, to be sure, relieving their symptoms as needed, and providing them existential comfort in their dying, but our intent can never be one that causes their death. It's not just that euthanasia provision counters good medicine; the biblical command not to take innocent life supersedes the request (Ex. 20:13; 2 Kgs. 21:16). Our primary mandate is to follow Christ, the Word incarnate, who said "if you love me, you will keep my commands" (John 14:15).

PROFESSIONALISM AND THE PROFESSION OF FAITH

This notion of a healthcare professional declining involvement in medical provision on the basis of conscience infringement goes against current sensibilities. In our era of secular humanism, such a stance is not only considered unacceptable, it's deemed *unprofessional*. This is due in part because of a general disregard for our past. Our culture suffers from a chronological snobbery, propping up the latest as the greatest, and holding in contempt our historical foundations. We've forgotten the wise words of Isaac Newton, who said with humility and respect, "If I have seen further it is by standing on the shoulders of giants."[16] The same can be said for the history of medicine. We have either carelessly forgotten or scornfully discarded the ground-breaking Christian legacy in Western healthcare provision.

The early church didn't just meet together on the Sabbath to worship and pray; they took their praises and thanksgiving into the streets, witnessing their faith in word and deed, including providing compassionate care for those in medical need. During the Cyprian Plague of the third Century, for example, Christians risked their lives in order to bring medical assistance and comfort to the diseased and dying. As the smallpox pandemic raged through Rome for two decades, killing hundreds by the day, the Christian community "showed unbounded love and loyalty, taking charge of the sick, ministering to them in Christ" while at the same time, the non-believers "pushed the sufferers away and even fled from their loved ones."[17] In addition to this acute response to medical crisis, the early church also acted as a long-term surrogate family for patients, providing cost-free care for both congregational members as well as outsiders. Following Christ's example, they welcomed those who were ill, and in so doing, reformed the prevalent view of sickness, and helped to destigmatize disease. While many healthcare institutions take pains to boast of their long-serving medical provision, it was the medieval Christian church that initially organized institutional healthcare provision, and established the first hospitals.[18] As well, the monasteries were the birthplace of nursing as a profession, and played a pivotal role in the holistic integration of spiritual and medical treatments, underscoring the importance of caring for the whole patient.

Medicine, understood as a caring profession, is fundamentally a Christian enterprise. The Christian worldview provides the only meaningful foundation for medical practice and the highest ethic of professionalism. Some may consider Hippocrates as having occupied this foundational position. And while there are many commendable points in his ancient pledge, such as the dedication to patient confidentiality and the opposition to both abortion and euthanasia, it wasn't until the Christian virtue of charity flourished that doctors were viewed as "good Samaritans motivated by altruism."[19] Unfortunately, this understanding of healthcare as a priestly calling has been largely dismissed. Rather, our role is being increasingly whittled down to that of base technician. As a result, the very understanding of what professionalism stands for has radically shifted. Not only has our Christian heritage been jettisoned from medical memory, but the ancient pillars of the Hippocratic Oath have also been pulled down. Despite the ethical guidance provided for over two millennia, these ancient tried-and-true virtues of medicine have been replaced by humanistic principles. Instead of extolling a physician's virtuous character and holding the practitioner accountable to the transcendent, present-day professionalism pays homage first and foremost to patient autonomy and non-paternalism. Accordingly, acting in a professional manner today is considered doing what you're told. Although lip service is still given to the adage, "first do no harm," neither killing the preborn nor injecting fatal drugs are considered such. "We don't need bleeding hearts and hand holders today," my medical director said; "It's researchers and technicians who'll take us to the next level of human evolution." Medicine has truly entered a *Dark Art* era. And as a result, a biblically faithful servanthood model may not only create potential conflicts within our doctor/patient relationships, but may also steer us headlong into combat with our medical regulating bodies and governance.

The provincial governing bodies of medicine in Canada have mandated that healthcare professionals dissociate their personal beliefs from their clinical obligations, including following the compass of conscience. For many physicians practicing in Canada, this isn't merely a potential conflict to be wary of, but a full-blown legal battle for conscience protection. Despite the fact that freedom of conscience has been enshrined in the *Canadian Charter of Rights & Freedoms* (Section 2), there remain provinces where conscience rights are in peril. Regulatory colleges can pass policies that require healthcare workers to refer for, and in some cases perform, physician-assisted suicide, whether or not the procedure goes against the practitioner's conscience. At the time of this writing, for example, in Ontario and Nova Scotia, doctors who refuse to perform MAID on moral grounds are being forced by their regulatory Colleges to refer patients for euthanasia, and coerced to be involved in violation of their moral convictions. This has jeopardized the medical practices of thousands of Ontario physicians, causing them to fear that they must choose between either their conscience or their careers. Despite the Ontario Divisional Court's pronouncement that these regulatory policies are in violation of the physicians' religious rights and freedoms, the requirements were felt to be justified because they ensured patient access to so-called healthcare.[20] In addition, advocates of euthanasia and physician-assisted suicide are intensely lobbying the government to force all publicly-funded healthcare facilities to offer assisted suicide on premises, even faith-based institutions, which have deeply-rooted principles that forbid them from directly ending the lives of their patients. In brief, conscientious objection seems to have lost its place in contemporary medicine.

So, why not just let up on the grace and truth tension at this point then? Perhaps we should forgo trying to defend scriptural truth, and just focus on getting along with everybody? After all, the apostle Paul even said that, "If it is possible, as far as it depends on you, live at peace with everyone" (Rom. 12:18). Isn't this possible? Can't we just get along... live and let live... don't rock the boat... and keep our noses clean? No doubt, such an approach applied to our professional sphere would likely ruffle less feathers with our peers or raise fewer eyebrows with our regulating bodies. But is that what Jesus would do in this situation? We mustn't forget about his whip made of cords to drive out the money changers, nor that he said, "Do you think that I have come to bring peace on earth? No, I tell you, but division" (Luke 12:51) – division from the earthly sinful ways that separate us from God. This Jesus-way tension is not an add-on topping to healthcare provision, like some kind of religious relish or Christian condiment. Rather, it's the very foundation of the feast, and one that lays claim to our professional lives. The maintenance of tension between Christ's exclusive claims and His inclusive compassion is an essential prerequisite for effectively living out our faith in the sphere of healthcare.

Before being executed for his part in the conspiracy to assassinate Adolf Hitler, Dietrich Bonhoeffer said, "When Christ calls a man, he bids him come and die."[21] If we are to bring reconciliation to medicine, we need to be prepared to take a stand on important issues, even if it means taking some flak. Scripture reminds us that "If you do not stand firm in your faith, you will not stand at all" (Is. 7:9). And as Jesus said, "Whoever wants to be my disciple must deny themselves and take up their cross and follow me" (Mark 8:43). Discipleship is less about us, and more about the Lord who calls us. So, as nice as it might be to lay low and not ruffle feathers, if we are to keep faith in medicine, complacency and compromise are not luxuries we can afford. There is a rich Christian heritage to the practice of Western healthcare, which we should be encouraged by. The torch has been passed to us, and now it's ours to carry high. After all, "God did not give us a spirit of timidity, but a spirit of power, of love and of self-discipline" (2 Tim. 1:7). Rather than viewing our work as merely a job, where we take on the title but neglect God's mandate, we need to see our work as a ministry where we co-labour with the Holy Spirit in the reconciliation of healthcare. In so doing, we move from medical practice as simply a vocation to medical practice as a witness and priestly calling. Our society is in desperate need of the salt and light of redemption. There are critical issues – like the ongoing abortion crisis, the acceptance of assisted suicide, the doomsday predictions of the environmental movement, and the sexualization of our culture – that are worth taking a stand against and resisting.

Some Perils of Going Public

When Jesus sent out his twelve disciples to the lost sheep of Israel, he did so with the warning to be "shrewd as snakes and as innocent as doves" (Matt. 10: 16), to which Preston Manning appended, "Not nasty as serpents and stupid as pigeons!" Certainly, getting involved in the public sphere as a Christian today can be fraught with danger. These are hostile times, so we need to proceed with caution. I've experienced this danger firsthand, and only too well recall the stomach-churning anguish of the experience.

It was in 2016, after the Alberta Education Minister, David Eggen, had implemented the gender diversity guidelines in our public schools.[22] Although presented under the pretense of creating safe spaces and a respectful environment for all children and teens, the recommendations were a clear promotion of LGBT ideology, and aimed at the deconstruction of sex, gender, and parenthood in our province. In the guidelines, for example, there was the encouragement for students to define their own gender (without their parents' involvement or knowledge), select their own personal pronoun, be permitted to play on either the boys or girls sports teams, have the option of using whichever change room or washroom they preferred, and to organize school-wide drag performances. In addition, there was a mandatory requirement for all students to take part in letter-writing campaigns advocating for LGBT rights, and for all schools to establish gay-straight alliance groups (GSAs). During this same time, the Alberta Teachers' Association rolled out their sexual education curriculum. Like the gender diversity guidelines, the updated sex-ed program had an indoctrination mandate targeting "every student, every class, every day." Teachers were given clear instructions to avoid using terms such as *boys and girls*, and instead use alternatives such as *comrades, folks,* and *friends*. Children as young as five years old were taught about the supposed spectrum of gender identity and gender

161

expression, as well as the diversity of emotional and sexual attractions available with wide ranging examples provided.

To make matters worse, sexually graphic material was being made available to public school children on government-funded websites. The Institute for Sexual Minority Studies and Services (iSMSS), hired by the provincial government to organize the Alberta Gay-Straight Alliance (GSA) Network, had online sexually explicit resources targeted at children aged 5-17 years of age. My wife and I were shocked to see what was accessible to school children with a simple click of a mouse: images of naked couples, including same-sex couples, details about various sexual positions, people being flogged and restrained, including instruction on how to use specific BDSM products (practices or roleplaying involving bondage, discipline, dominance and submission, sadomasochism), as well as purchasing instructions. Masturbation clubs were advertised with encouragements to "pay for porn" and to "visit a group masturbation night at your local sex club." It was indecent and irresponsible, and I felt that an urgent response was needed – not only as a parent with school-aged children, but as a physician, aware of the harmful and addictive impact of pornographic images on the developing brain, and as a Christian, understanding the demonic nature of sexual idolatry.

Together with a fellow medical colleague, I responded by writing a paper to the Education Minister, in which we detailed medically-based concerns with his gender diversity recommendations. Our document was made public with its simultaneous posting on the *Parents for Choice* website (an Alberta-based, non-profit advocacy organization encouraging excellence in education through parental participation).[23] Within days, we received a flurry of both positive and negative responses to our written concerns. On the positive side, numerous parents contacted us with their praise for our reasoned arguments and encouragement for our bold counter to the government's foisted recommendations. Many were not aware of the complexity of the issues at hand, and were pleased to have a medical voice added to their own concerns. Although we didn't receive any formal response from the Education Minister, enough pressure had been placed on his office by concerned parents that the graphic material, which had been on the government-sponsored websites, ended up being removed. Of course, it wasn't all laurels and hearty handshakes. There were also the negative responses that we received. Although the criticisms were less in number, they were packed full of vehement anger and accusations. Rather than critiquing our posed arguments, the negative responders made use of ad hominem attacks, accusing us of being "ignorant," "homophobic," and "transphobic." The College of Physicians and Surgeons also sent me a formal complaint, initiated by one of the students, reprimanding me for my part in the letter, and warning me not to repeat such a misdeed. As a whole, it was difficult reading, and conjured feelings of vulnerability and fear.

When we thought the worst might be over, it came to our attention that an online petition had been launched against us. It was signed by over one hundred medical students, denouncing our article, trouncing our reputations, and calling for our immediate removal from the University. Numerous emails and phone calls transpired, including lengthy discussions with University department heads and the Dean of Medicine. The resultant anguish drove me to my knees. As the pressures mounted and our professional careers seemed to hang in the balance, I found myself reading my Bible more frequently and with more intention. My prayer life intensified, and my morning devotions lengthened. The Sermon on the Mount spoke to me anew, and brought clarity to my situation and comfort to my distress: "Blessed are those who are persecuted because of righteousness, for theirs is the kingdom of heaven" (Matt. 5:10).

The debacle finally came to a head when the Dean held a special meeting to discuss the situation. Medical students from all years were invited to attend, as were numerous faculty members. Despite feeling anxious about the outcome, I was deeply pleased and proud to hear that a number of Christian medical students, whom my colleague and I had separately mentored over the years, stood up bravely in front of their peers to defend our characters and views. And fortunately for us, cool heads prevailed. In the end, we didn't have to rescind our University credentialing. We were reprimanded for not having a disclaimer on our article, and instructed to promptly add one, making clear to readers that the views expressed were ours and not the position of the University. As for the students involved in our social media smear campaign, they were rebuked for their methods, and instructed to take down their online comments.

This disquieting experience made real to me the danger that Christians can face when speaking out in the public sphere on controversial issues. While this may be unavoidable at times, it's important to realize that this doesn't always have to be the case. Pushing back against societal distortions and decay doesn't necessarily need to result in the kind of crossfire exposure we experienced. There are plenty of ways one can be meaningfully involved in Kingdom work without ending up in the crosshairs. Online advocacy support for *Informed Albertans* and the *Parents for Choice in Education* organization were largely responsible for the eventual removal of the sexually graphic material from the provincial government's school website. The key is that we work together as a Christian community. The leftist groups are extremely well-organized in this respect, and can rapidly mobilize through social media to push their agenda. In order to reform culture with gospel truth, we have to follow suit and ensure that our voice is also heard. Keeping informed of the issues and promptly signing online petitions are safe and simple ways of reforming culture that we can all be involved with.

Additionally, we can engage the hot-button issues of our day without feeling the heat by supporting Christian parachurch organizations. Encouragement, prayer, volunteer hours, and financial support for such organizations, positioned on the frontlines of cultural battle, can go a long ways in the reconciliation of our society. One can help defend our Constitutional freedoms, for example, by providing a donation to the *Justice Centre for Constitutional Freedoms*, or assist in the lobby against euthanasia by becoming a member of the *Euthanasia Prevention Coalition*. We can help realize the vision of enhanced Christian leadership in our society by becoming a builder with *the Ezra Institute for Contemporary Christianity*. By supporting their young adult high-impact training programs, we can help reform our culture by ensuring that the gospel message be proclaimed to the next generation. We need to be careful, to be sure, but not complacent.

CONCLUDING REMARKS

The message of God's reconciliation is an all-encompassing one. Every sphere of our culture is to be redeemed and no portion left exempt. Our efforts with the Holy Spirit are not to be restricted to the confines of the church, nor to our private devotions, but need to broadly engage every aspect of our lives. As the psalmist proclaims, "The earth is the Lord's, and everything in it" (Ps. 24:1). Considered in this way, the scope of God's reconciliation for the world is as great as that of the fall. Just as the whole of creation was affected by the fall, so too, the whole of creation is to be reconciled, including our public involvement, our family life, and the practice of medicine. As Albert Wolters asserts, "part of God's plan for the earth is that it be filled and subdued by humankind; that its latent possibilities be unlocked and actualized in human history and civilization."[24] So, rather than trying to turn the hands of the clock backwards, to return to some form of Eden, the ministry of reconciliation points forward to a new Heaven and earth. In his *Letter from Birmingham Jail*, Dr. Martin Luther King Jr., wrote, "There was a time when the church was very powerful – in the time when the early Christians rejoiced at being deemed worthy to suffer for what they believed. In those days the church was not merely a thermometer that recorded the ideas and principles of popular opinion; it was a thermostat that transformed the mores of society..."[25] If we are to keep our faith in medicine, we need to be thermostats rather than thermometers, and actively involved in these reconciliation efforts. This means living out our faith in word and deed on a daily basis – in the clinic, the emergency room, the surgical suite, on the ward – wherever we've been planted, and whatever the costs may be.

SUMMARY POINTS – RECONCILIATION

1. God has invited us to co-labour with the Holy Spirit in His all-encompassing ministry of reconciliation

2. The cultural narrative of neutrality creates an artificial distinction between sacred and secular realms, compartmentalizing and secularizing our lives

3. Sabbath-keeping and daily praise and thanksgiving can help to protect us from the secularization of healthcare provision

4. An attitude of servanthood allows us to maintain the tension between Christ's exclusive claims and His inclusive care and compassion

5. The priestly role of medicine is at odds with contemporary medical governance and may generate conflict in our practice

6. Considering our patients as neighbors to whom we are called to love, we will need to sometimes disagree with them and allow them to pursue their intentions without our cooperation

7. The Christian heritage of medicine is responsible for our current Western medicine model and success

Questions for Reflection and Discussion

1.   Do you agree that there is no neutral ground? Why or why not? What evidence would you give to support your perspective?

2.   Have you also struggled with secularization or the sacred/secular divide? What helped you deal with this?

3.   Is Sabbath-keeping part of your Christian life? Was there a time when it was or wasn't?

4.   Why is the Sabbath important to you? How could you further develop the Sabbath as a spiritual discipline?

5.   What role does praise have in your Christian life? Do you have a favorite song or praise or a particular praise memory?

6.   How important is gratitude in your life? Do you *give thanks* for your meal when you're at a restaurant, or outside your regular home environment?

7.   Why is it important to think in terms of mission field? Where do you see your current mission field? Was there a time when you had a different mission field? Where was it?

8.   As we consider the tension between biblical truth and compassionate care, have you been too far on one side of the spectrum or the other? Overly condemning... overly affirming? What steps could you take to better maintain the needed balance?

9.   Are patients neighbors in the biblical sense? How do we best show our love for them?

10. How would you respond to a patient who requested referral for

gender reassignment? An abortion? MAID?

11. Is reconciliation an achievable goal? How can we be involved in our professional sphere? The public sphere? Our personal sphere of influence?

CHAPTER NOTES

1. Stout, Jeffrey. *Ethics after Babel: the Languages of Morals and Their Discontents.* Princeton: Princeton University Press, 2001.

2. Peterson, Eugene. *Christ Plays in Ten Thousand Places: a Conversation in Spiritual Theology.* Eerdmans, 2008.

3. Chambers, Oswald. *Utmost Classic Readings and Prayers from Oswald Chambers: 90 Days of Inspirational Reading to Strengthen Your Soul.* Oswald Chambers Publications, 2012.

4. Carretto, Carlo. *The God Who Comes.* Darton, Longman & Todd, 1974.

5. Dallas, Joe, and Heche, Nancy. *The Complete Christian Guide to Understanding Homosexuality: a Biblical and Compassionate Response to Same-sex Attraction.* Harvest House Publishers, 2010.

6. Robles, H. *Reverence for Life: The Words of Albert Schweitzer.* Harper Collins 1993.

7. Ratcliffe, S. *Oxford Essential Quotations* (4 ed.) 2016 Oxford University Press.

8. Peterson, Eugene. *The Jesus Way: a Conversation of the Ways Jesus is the Way.* Eerdmans, 2007.

9. MacDonald, George. *Life Essential: the hope of the Gospel.* Regent College Publishing. 2004.

10. Dickens, Charles. *A Christmas Carol.* Penguin, 2014.

11. Mayer, Lawrence, and McHugh, Paul. "Sexuality and Gender: Findings from the Biological, Psychological, and Social Sciences." *The New Atlantis* (Special Report). August 2016, http://www.thenewatlantis.com/publications/number-50-fall-2016.

12. Moore, E., Wisniewski, A. and Dobs, A. "Endocrine treatment of transsexual people: A review of treatment regimens, outcomes, and adverse effects." *The Journal of Endocrinology & Metabolism,* 2003;88(9):3467-3473.

13. Yarhouse, Mark. *Understanding Gender Dysphoria: Navigating Transgender Issues in a Changing Culture.* InterVarsity Press, 2015.

14. See for example, Physicians for Life: https://www.physiciansforlife.ca/

15. The Back Porch: http://www.thebackporch.info

16. Newton, Isaac. "Letter from Sir Isaac Newton to Robert Hooke." *Historical Society of Pennsylvania.*

17. Williamson, G.A. *The History of the Church: From Christ to Constantine.* Penguin, 1989.

18. Ferngren, Gary B. *Medicine & Health Care in Early Christianity*, Johns Hopkins University Press, 2009.

19. Porter, Roy. *The Greatest Benefit to Mankind: A Medical History of Humanity.* W.W. Norton 1999.

20. Christian Medical and Dental Society of Canada v. College of Physicians and Surgeons of Ontario, 2018 ONSC 579.

21. Bonhoeffer, Dietrich. *The Cost of Discipleship. Touchstone, 1995.*

22. "Guidelines for Best Practices: Creating Learning Environments that respect Diverse Sexual Orientations, Gender Identities and Gender Expressions." *Government of Alberta*, 2016. https://education.alberta.ca/media/1626737/91383-attachment-1-guidelines-final.pdf.

23. Achen, Blaine, and Fenske, Theodore K. "A Medical Response to Alberta Education's Gender Diversity: Guidelines for Best Practices." *Parent Choice*, 2016. https://www.parentchoice.ca/a_medical_response_to_alberta_educations_gender_diversity_guidelines_for_best_practices

24. Wolters, Albert. *Creation Regained: Biblical Basics for a Reformational Worldview.* Eerdmans Publishing Co. 1985.

25. King, Jr. M. "Letter from a Birmingham Jail," April 16, 1963. Hosted at University of Pennsylvania – African Studies Center. https://www.africa.upenn.edu/Articles_Gen/Letter_Birmingham.html.

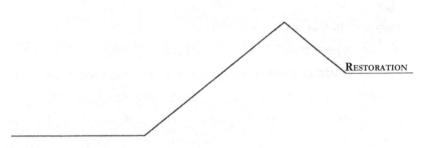

CHAPTER 5

DENIAL AND DEFEAT

"I know that my redeemer lives, and that in the end he will stand on
the earth. And after my skin has been destroyed, yet in my flesh I will
see God; I myself will see him with my own eyes –
I, and not another."
Job 19:25-17

THE BLEAK HERE AND NOW

The gospel contour concludes with triumphant *Restoration*. As twisted,
misdirected, and distorted as things have become on our troubled terra
firma, Scripture provides clear assurance that everything will be made
good again in the fullness of time. The Bible emphasizes that the chal-

173

lenges of our present circumstances are but temporary. We are given reason to anticipate a place where the bonds of servitude will be broken, and evil oppression will end, where righteous judgement will be delivered, and all crimes see perfect justice, and a time when selfish ambition and sexual temptation will cease. Although foreign to our earthly experiences, we are told that what awaits us is "a new Heaven and a new earth… where there will be no more death or mourning or crying or pain, for the old order of things has passed away" (Rev. 21:1-4). It's an ultimate wrap-up that has inspired countless generations of Christians to fight the good fight, finish the race, and keep the faith (2 Tim. 4:7).

The take-home message of Christian eschatology is that there's *more* to life than our experience of the physical world, and *more* to death than the decay of our physical bodies. It's important to realize that this *more* isn't something we just need to wait patiently for, as "pie in the sky when we die, by and by." This *more* starts right here and right now. Scripture claims that "the Kingdom is in our midst" (Luke 17:21). Jesus clarified this by saying, "Now this is eternal life: that they know you, the only true God, and Jesus Christ, whom you have sent "(John 17:3). As a result of God's incarnation, and the personal relationship that He offers each of us, we can experience certain aspects of eternal life in our present moments. By submitting ourselves to God's will and immersing ourselves in intimate relationship with the living Christ, we can participate in the ushering in of this gospel resolution, and lay claim to our citizenship in Heaven (Phil. 3:20). It's a game-changing revelation which confirms that our suffering has meaning and that our work has purpose.

Our contemporary culture dismisses biblical eschatology as either nursery-room whimsy, or naive wishful thinking. Saturated in materialism, the prevailing view of our culture holds fast to a bleak *here-and-now* understanding of life, and an even bleaker *too-bad-so-sad* outlook on death. John Lennon's signature song, *Imagine*, popularized this secular sentiment in the '70s, and continues to have an influence today. Although the winsome melody and call to solidarity are attractive – "Imagine there's no Heaven; It's easy if you try; No Hell below us; above us, only sky" – his empty words betray the ultimate hopelessness of Lennon's worldview. If all we have is the here and now, then all we have is without eternal meaning or purpose. Adding to this, such a surface-level material view of reality places pressure on our present moments. By attempting to skirt divine judgement, and eliminate binding morality, this perspective necessitates that Heaven and Hell – in some sense – get worked out in our lifetimes. This means that we are forced to chase after some form of plastic paradise, and simultaneously avenge ourselves of the wrongs others have done to us. Those who hold to this impoverished worldview are left to madly check off items from their bucket list in search of illusive happiness and desperately seek immediate vengeance for wrongs they've endured. As William Ralph Inge wisely observed, "We can only say that secularism, like other religions, needs an eschatology, and has produced one."

Medical culture is inundated with *here and now* thinking, as well. Although there has been a recent rise in paganism and an ongoing fascination with Eastern mysticism, the superficial adherence to these amorphous spiritualties by a large proportion or our society isn't given much serious consideration in the empirical world of healthcare. In the messy science of medicine, life is understood from *'just the facts'* and is quickly reduced to a *'what you see is what you get'* experience. There's work to be done, after all, and no time to be wasted on things without a tangible evidential base. As for death, it's generally regarded as a defeat. Our primary efforts are focussed on countering it, avoiding it, delaying it, and even attempting to reverse it. So, when death finally arrives and stakes its territory, we generally accept it as the ultimate of all failings and finalities, and limp onward. Marlene Dietrich, the long-lived German-American star of classic Hollywood cinema, bluntly summed this up by saying, "When you're dead, you're dead. That's it." A bankrupt philosophy, to be sure, but one that has been readily adopted by those in healthcare. We see so much death in our work week; it's easy to get numb to it all. When the 'code blue' is finally called, and we draw the blanket over the face of the deceased, there's no denying the quiet finality that pervades the post-resuscitation clean-up, and no escaping the overwhelming feeling that death has won, and we have lost.

WHAT'S A HEAVEN FOR?

Even though I managed to maintain a Christian perspective in most aspects of my life, I struggled for the longest time with the Restoration portion of the gospel narrative. Despite growing up in the church and weekly reciting the Apostle's Creed – "I believe in the Holy Spirit... the resurrection of the body, and life everlasting" – Christian eschatology remained a formidable challenge for me to accept. Judgement aside, it all seemed too good to be true. The promise of eternal destiny, and all those ideas around end times, Heaven and Hell... just seemed like wishful thinking. It wasn't that I'd been sheltered from end-of-life considerations. I was no stranger to the specter of death – far from it, in fact. Long before medical school, I experienced its ugly harshness. During my high school graduating year, I was thrust head-first into the turmoil and grief of the dying process when my mother was diagnosed with terminal cancer. Comforting her through her exhausting bouts of chemotherapy was often overwhelming. Although I initially tried to deny that her condition was serious, as the weeks passed and her condition worsened, my stubborn denial turned to angry demands.

"Why can't more be done?" I'd ask my shell-shocked father. "What about bone marrow transplantation… or sending her to the Mayo Clinic?!"

As months wore on and her Irish beauty was slowly stripped away, eventually leaving behind a hardly recognizable shadow of my mother, these earlier demands gave way to requests of despair.

"Take me, instead, Lord," I would pray. "Please take me, instead," I repeated, as I cried myself to sleep most nights.

I recall my overwhelming feelings of fear as her death drew near, and the raw anguish as we prepared to lose her. When she died, I found certain solace in Scripture, and was comforted by the idea that death was not the end and that eternal life awaited her. I longed to believe this, mainly because the thought of her not existing was unbearable for me. So, for my mother's sake, if for no other reason, I was determined to hold on to some version of the Christian eschatology of Heaven. Yet as the years passed, and moss grew over her gravestone, this determination weakened. As the engraved letters on her nameplate faded, so did my youthful belief in the afterlife. I had a growing fear that perhaps Marlene Dietrich was right. Maybe she was just "dead. That's it." I began to suspect that there was no Heaven, after all, and wondered if her only real afterlife might be the memories that she had left behind. Like the pastor portrayed by Greg Kinnear in the movie, "Heaven is for Real," I began to second guess the reality of everlasting life.

During my medical training years, my doubts about Heaven and the afterlife only increased. As a cardiology resident, I saw a great deal of death. During my role as Code Captain, this was particularly the case. I was responsible for running all the cardiac arrest "codes" that occurred throughout the hospital while on call, and was thrust regularly into the dramatic struggle between life and death. Sometimes the emergency calls would come back to back, with only brief moments between them to restock the code cart. Occasionally, more than one stat page would ring out simultaneously, creating a certain logistical challenge and triage nightmare. At times, I felt a bit like the Grim Reaper's bellboy, running up and down the hospital hallways at all hours, pronouncing death and delivering news of despair. And in the end it was always the same. When patients died, they stayed dead – even the successfully resuscitated ones eventually died. The idea of life after death seemed far removed from my reality.

While I retained a Christian confession to an extent, the recurring experiences of death and despair hardened my heart and rendered my thinking more and more that of a humanist. My thoughts of the afterlife took on a metaphorical and pragmatic understanding. The words of Robert Browning, the English poet, rang true to me when he wrote, "A man's reach should exceed his grasp; or what's a Heaven for?" At that time, I considered Heaven to be a human construct. I figured that it functioned as an incentive for self-improvement. Just as dreams were important for achievements and imagination for understanding, so I considered Heaven helpful for self-actualization. Rather than envisioning Heaven as laid out in the book of Revelation, I thought of it as an illusionary Olympic carrot, encouraging us ever "faster, higher, stronger."

It wasn't until after my first year as a staff cardiologist that these secularized conceptualizations of the afterlife were challenged. I was on conference leave with my wife and young family in the United States when I heard the tragic news of the ill-fated Swissair Flight 111. The plane crash claimed all 229 lives on board as it hit the waters off the shores of Nova Scotia near Peggy's Cove. Although I was aware of many other such tragedies over the years, this one really struck home. I was born in Halifax, I knew the area well, and had countless memories of clambering over the rocks along that coastline during family picnics beside the Peggy's Point Lighthouse. The horrifying televised images of the debris field, all covered in jet fuel, and with body parts floating amid pieces of the plane wreckage, made me sick to my stomach. Although I was relatively young and fit, was happily married with healthy children, and still had my whole bright-shiny career before me, the disaster shook me to the core, as it forced me to consider my own mortality.

My figurative concept of Heaven was insufficient to be of any comfort and of limited value to help me come to terms with such a tragedy. It was then that I realized my understanding of the gospel was incomplete, and that I was ill-prepared to face the sting of death. It dawned on me that even though I knew that I was a child of God, and that He would not abandon me in suffering, and had saved me from my sins... there was more. I also needed to be sure of His eternal plan for me, and that only then would the gospel have its full redeeming power in my life. In brief, I realized that Heaven couldn't wait, but needed to be seriously addressed and biblically understood.

Years later I had a chance to visit the two Swissair Memorials along the Lighthouse Way in Nova Scotia, and grieve once again over the tragic loss. It was during that time that I attended a men's retreat and experienced a Heaven-clarifying realization. The theme of the retreat was developing spiritual disciplines. Incorporated into the weekend were a series of activities designed to provide us attendees with some practical opportunities to apply what we'd learned. One such activity was aimed to cultivate our appreciation for solitary reflection. During this half-hour exercise, we were instructed to take a slip of paper from a basket being passed around, find a quiet place, and reflect and pray on the slip's printed Scripture verse. After taking my slip from the basket, I made off for a quiet spot to pray. However, it was difficult finding a spot; each area I arrived at was already occupied by one of the other men. With time running out, I quickened my pace and happened upon a small secluded graveyard, complete with park bench. Having found the perfect spot, I sat among the gravestones, and pulled out my slip of paper which read, "I am alive with Christ" (Eph. 2:5). I smiled to myself and thought, "Here I am alive with Christ, surrounded by all these dead bodies…" Then, as I tried to get past the irony of the situation and focus on the Scripture slip, the words of Jesus came to mind, "I am the resurrection and the life. The one who believes in me will live, even though they die" (John 11:25). As I sat quietly, it occurred to me that perhaps I wasn't the only one *alive in Christ* in the cemetery. Although I was still physically alone there amongst the gravestones, it dawned on me that all those who had followed Christ, even though they had died and were buried about me, were also *alive with Christ*, as well. I further realized that being *alive with Christ* was independent of biological life. If I was *alive with Christ*, while sitting there on the cemetery bench with heart beating and neurons firing, I would remain so even after my own gravestone got moss-covered and forgotten, and for all eternity beyond that. As I prayed there amongst the tombstones, the Swissair memorial was brought to my mind. The truth that those believers who perished that day are also alive in Christ provided some genuine consolation. Then the answer to Robert Browning's rhetorical question – "What's a Heaven is for?" – became clear to me; "Heaven is for real!"

The Whole Truth and Nothing but the Truth

To keep our faith in the centre of our medical profession – including our end-of-life care – it's important to have a biblically faithful understanding of death and the afterlife. Heaven can't wait for some future epiphany. Our eternal destiny promised in the Bible needs to be rightly understood within the context of the entire gospel narrative. To protect ourselves from reducing certain portions of the Bible to something lesser – particularly the more difficult passages or doctrines, like Heaven, Hell, and judgement – we need to maintain a high view of Scripture, a view that supersedes all incoming secular thoughts and ideas. As the apostle Paul warns, "See to it that no one takes you captive through hollow and deceptive philosophy, which depends on human tradition and the elemental spiritual forces of this world rather than on Christ" (Col. 2:8). To do so, it's important to recognize the Bible as the ultimate authority, and appreciate its all-sufficient foundational explanatory power.

The Bible isn't just a source for devotional comfort and Sunday inspiration, nor a list of moral platitudes. It's also not simply a series of worldview prooftexts for use in arguments, nor a book of personal preferences that we can pick and choose from like someone selecting food at a buffet. The Bible can't be broken up into bits and bites and simply utilized in some fragmentary fashion. While we can make use of individual Scripture passages at times, such as my Scripture scripts, it's important to keep in mind their context, and consider them in the entirety of the Word. The gospel shouldn't be reduced to the one-liner, "Jesus died for our sins," nor confined to the first four books of the newer Testament. While the gospel emphasizes Christ's redemption and is detailed in the accounts of Matthew, Mark, Luke and John, it's better to consider it as a single, unified, unfolding and progressive grand narrative woven throughout the Bible, older and newer Testaments. While the biblical Canon represents a collection of 66 books written by 40 inspired authors from different cultural and geographic contexts, and spanning two millennia, it can only be properly understood and faithfully followed if considered as a complete unity. This *trans-biblical* gospel message uses a single voice, and holds together as a unity with no one portion able to stand alone without the other. It's a take-it-or-leave-it, all-or-none package that we need to accept in its entirety, and as it's been faithfully passed down to us.

One practical approach that I have found useful to accentuate and develop this appreciation of the Bible as a complete unity is to make regular use of the cross-reference feature in the text margins while reading Scripture. Understanding how certain themes or verses recur in different parts of the Bible has given me a better appreciation of the one voice that weaves throughout Scripture. For example, consider the unfavorable offering of Cain in Genesis 4:5, and how this is developed by Samuel in his rhetorical rebuke, "Does the Lord delight in burnt offerings and sacrifices as much as in obeying the voice of the Lord?" Then this concern of God's is set as an imperative in the Psalms with "Offer right sacrifices" (Ps. 4:5), and underscored by Solomon in the Wisdom literature with "To do what is right and just is more acceptable to the Lord than sacrifice" (Prov. 21:3). The prophet Hosea emphasizes this further by saying, "I desire mercy not sacrifice" (Hos. 6:6). Jesus places this quote into the context of salvation by saying, "It is not the healthy who need a doctor, but those who are ill. But go and learn what this means: 'I desire mercy, not sacrifice.' For I have not come to call the righteous, but sinners" (Matt. 9:12-14).

The Bible as Ultimate Commitment

My intent is not an erudite lesson in hermeneutics or biblical exegesis, but simply to emphasize that the Bible makes most sense when treated as a complete unity. Cross-references like these not only add depth and colour to biblical interpretation, they illustrate the connections between the various books of Scripture, and help to conceptually tie the Bible together as a cohesive whole. This is important since, taken as a complete work, the Bible represents the objectively true account of reality, and is our foundation for knowing things, and how we know them, as well as our authoritative moral standard. In essence, the biblical worldview is how we make sense of the world. And not just the world in religious terms or church context, but in all terms and every context – scientific, medical, ethical, legal, and educational, as well as the sphere of the intangible. While Scripture wasn't intended to be exhaustive in content, it does stand as an authoritative foundation for how all things are rightly understood. It's critical to understand this, because "If the foundations are destroyed, what can the righteous do?" (Ps. 11:3).

In matters of science, for example, the Bible provides the preconditions necessary for the uniformity of nature. It is God's providential and sovereign governance of the universe that affords the necessary conditions for scientific experimentation, including the inexact science of medical practice. Because "God is not a God of disorder" (1 Cor. 14:33), we can do science. Without the divine uniformity of nature, there would be no way of predicting the result of any given action. Random actions would merely produce random results, different every time. As a result, not a single experiment would be possible, and not a single medical prescription meaningful.

In the sphere of ethics, the Bible provides the absolute standard to measure good from bad and right from wrong. Without a transcendent reference point, morality becomes a mere human construction and quickly breaks down into little more than whim and fancy, and my liking or your preference. As C. S. Lewis pointed out, "A man does not call a line crooked unless he has some idea of a straight line."[1]

Likewise, the Bible gives grounding for law. This is the case not only for jurisprudence, but for all forms of law, including the physical laws of nature and the laws of logic. In regard to the laws of mathematics, reformed theologian and philosopher Cornelius Van Til said, "Atheists may be able to count... but they can't account for their counting without God." To be meaningful, abstract entities like numbers and thought progressions need God as their immaterial reference point and provider of meaning. This is the case since behind all law is necessarily the doctrine of sovereignty, which can only be justifiably supplied by the

Sovereign King of the universe. As the prophets declared, "I will put my law within them, and I will write it on their hearts. And I will be their God, and they shall be my people" (Jer. 31:33).

Additionally, the Bible is the foundation for all education, knowledge and learning. Factual knowledge isn't composed of isolated facts in a vacuum. Every fact must be connected to other facts in order to be comprehensible. And to be meaningful, all facts must ultimately be in relationship to the absolute, personal God of Scripture, who governs all things and gives them meaning. The facts that allow for knowledge, learning, and education can only do so because of their relationship to the revealed God of Scripture. As the apostle Paul proclaims, "no man can lay a foundation other than the one which is laid, which is Jesus Christ" (1 Cor. 3:11).

The all-important intangibles like thoughts and imagination also can't exist by floating in the physical realm, but require an intellectual mooring. They, too, depend upon a biblical foundation to be anything more than mere human fabrications. How can immaterial realities like hope, beauty, and dignity have a meaningful explanation in a solely materialistic worldview of matter in motion? Only the personal triune God revealed in the Bible can provide the necessary underpinning for these and give them meaning. As detailed in Scripture, the virtues of "love, joy, peace, forbearance, kindness, goodness, faithfulness, gentleness and self-control" are nothing less than manifested fruit of the Holy Spirit (Gal. 5:22-23).

While secular thinkers may claim that God isn't necessary for any scientific endeavor or immaterial ideation, this is because they unwittingly operate on Christian real estate. They carry on in ignorant branches of bliss without acknowledging God as the root and trunk of the tree of life. As theologian and apologist Greg Bahnsen summarized, "the Christian worldview is not only the only hope of future salvation;

184

it's our only present intellectual hope."[2] It's become clear to me that since the full-blown gospel message in all its entirety is required to make sense of our world and experiences, every portion of the gospel message is important. No part can be excluded, even the passages that are difficult to accept or understand. So, despite the challenges that eternal resolution posed for me in the past, and the mystery it still presents, I choose to accept God's eternal promises because then, and only then, can I make sense of the full gamut of my experiences. Like Saint Augustine of Hippo who said, "I believe in order to understand," I believe Heaven to be true in order to understand the meaning and purpose in our world. It no longer bothers me that, as a physician, I can't fathom the resurrection of the body. Since, truth be told, there's no shortage of things I can't fathom. (I don't really know how my laptop works, or even my toaster oven for that matter). So, why should I be fussed over eternal mysteries? Like the psalmist, then, "I do not concern myself with great matters or things too wonderful for me. But I have calmed and quieted myself… like a weaned child I am content" (Ps. 131:1-2).

THE SPIRITUAL DISCIPLINE OF FASTING

To help protect ourselves from falling prey to secular thought and adopting an impoverished understanding of our lives and mortality, we need to keep ever focussed on the gospel message in its entirety. Spiritual disciplines engender this needed focus, and of them, *fasting* is perhaps the most effective. Shared by many of the world religions, self-denial through fasting is widely recognized as a central means of achieving spiritual clarity and intimacy with God. As William Law, the eighteenth-century Church of England priest wisely said, "If religion requires us sometimes to fast and to deny our natural appetites, it is to lessen that struggle and war that is in our nature. It is to render our bodies fitter instruments of purity and more obedient to the good motions of divine grace. It is to dry up the springs of our passions that war against the soul, to cool the flame of our blood, and to render the mind more capable of divine meditations."[3] Although fasting has been described as the most neglected of the spiritual disciplines, its practice and value are emphasized throughout Scripture.[4] Moses fasted for 40 days prior to receiving the Ten Commandments (Ex. 34:28), as did Jesus before facing his pre-ministry temptation (Luke 4:2-4). And as an intentional counter to our material-minded consumer culture, I can think of no better form of protection.

My first experience with fasting was on medical mission in the Congo during the Rwandan genocide. It wasn't a self-imposed spiritual discipline of piety by any means, but rather a situation-imposed endurance of necessity. Our medical team was lodged at a resource-limited compound provided by one of the local churches. As it turned out, breakfast and lunch were among those limitations and were not offered. I learned this the hard way. After my early morning jog to rev up my metabolic engine, I went into the compound kitchen to fill up my gastric tank. But like the nursery rhyme of old Mother Hubbard, who went to the cupboard, to give the poor dog a bone, when I got there, the cupboard was bare, and I was the one who had none. So, with stomach grumbling, I joined the rest of the hungry team as we made our long morning commute to the Kibumba refugee camp. As per the adage, *misery loves company*, we at least had each other, as well as access to plenty of fluids. Formerly the Belgian Congo, the locals were able to offer us strong Belgian-styled espresso, which we imbibed along with copious amounts of bottled water. While warmth and hydration provided a base level of comfort, we were constantly reminded of our calorie-free state by the intermittent gnawing pains in our stomachs, and commiserated with each other by exchanging pained facial expressions and muttered complaints. Although the busy clinic served as a certain distraction from the unwanted fasting, my empty stomach remained in the forefront of my mind, and was joined by feelings of anxiety and even fear. As the day progressed, my stomach grumbling developed into audible gurgling, as did the bellies of my colleagues. By the time we packed up our supplies and got loaded into the vehicle, we had a battle of the borborygmi bands playing for the entire return trip to the compound.

After that early negative experience, I've since come to appreciate the tremendous benefits from self-imposed fasting, both as a spiritual discipline, as well as a weight control measure. Working alongside dieticians in the cardiovascular risk reduction clinic, I've learned about the pros and cons of various popular diets and therapeutic weight-control interventions. Intermittent fasting is the most effective of these interventions, and has been proven to offset the metabolic syndrome and improve body composition for patients with excessive abdominal fat.[5]

My own experience corroborates this. In addition to a prudent diet and exercise regimen, incorporating two to three 16-hour intermittent fasts into my work week has allowed me to successfully maintain an ideal body weight and prevent the commonly experienced dilemma of middle age – *when your age starts showing around your middle.* I begin my fast after a bowl of granola and milk before retiring to bed, accomplishing the first portion of my fasting state while sleeping. Then on waking, I drink a tall glass of water, and sip on a doppio espresso during my morning devotional. Freed up from meal preparation, I have extra time to reflect on Scripture, and I make a point of choosing a specific prayer request for the day. From a leadership appeal for our student CMDA chapter, to an appeal for comfort and consolation for a dying friend, I lay out my prayer request before the Lord, and allow my grumbling stomach to keep it in the forefront of my mind. Then with numerous bottles of water and a large thermos of plain tea, I take on the business of my day, fueled by Scripture and filled with the Spirit. After my clinic is finished in late afternoon, I break my fasting state with a cup of beef broth, followed by a small packed lunch meal, and do so with intensified gratitude for God's caloric provisions. Food never tasted better.

Fasting is a powerful reminder of our mortality and dependence on God. When we are physically outside of our comfort zone, we can become more aware of God's presence in our lives. When Jesus was tempted with food after his prolonged fast, he quoted from the Torah, "man does not live on bread alone but on every word that comes from the mouth of the Lord" (Deut. 8:3). While man doesn't live long without bread, either, the intermittent hunger pangs produced by the fasting state allow us to hear God's voice all the clearer. As C. S. Lewis said, "Pain insists upon being attended to. God whispers to us in our pleasures, speaks in our consciences, but shouts in our pains." So, during my fast, instead of perseverating on how hungry I feel, I reflect on the satisfaction of being God's child. My growling stomach brings to mind Isaiah's analogy of the Lord Almighty "as a lion growls, a great lion over its prey" (Isa. 31:4). By using my hunger pangs as a prompt to consider the Scripture passages and recall my prayer request, they become easily bearable. I don't announce my fast days to anyone, but keep the experience a private matter between myself and the Lord. As Jesus commanded, "when you fast, put oil on your head and wash your face, so that it will not be obvious to others that you are fasting, but only to your Father, who is unseen; and your Father, who sees what is done in secret, will reward you" (Matt. 6:17). In this way, I take the fasting experience beyond a biological weight-control exercise, and link the fat-burning benefits to the spiritual discipline of self-denial. My stomach emptiness reminds me of God's fullness; and my poverty in His abundance.

SHARING OUR TEST-A-MINUTE

To help keep a full-orbed gospel understanding in mind, I wear a purple cloth wrist band with the embroidered phrase, "HE IS RISEN!" in white letters. It serves as a moment-by-moment tangible reminder of the importance of Christ's historical resurrection and God's planned triumphant and complete restoration of all things, including my own bodily resurrection. As the apostle Paul said, "if the dead are not raised, then Christ has not been raised either. And if Christ has not been raised, your faith is futile; you are still in your sins. Then those also who have fallen asleep in Christ are lost. If only for this life we have hope in Christ, we are of all people most to be pitied" (1 Cor. 15:16-19). The strap and letters are easily visible next to my Timex and gospel bracelet, and sometimes garner the attention of those around me, including my patients and students. If asked, I share something of my faith and struggle. So despite the fact the ends are a bit frayed and tattered, I continue to faithfully wear the wrist band, and do so for two reasons. First and foremost, it functions as a personal reminder of my eternal destiny. And secondly, wearing it visible on my wrist affords opportunities to share certain aspects of my faith with others. While this sort of sharing might be frowned upon by the purveyors of medical education, there is definite merit in developing comfort in talking about certain aspects of our stories with patients, including our faith stories. Even though Christianity isn't popular in our culture, we must not be ashamed, since as the apostle Paul reminds us, "(the gospel) is the power of God that brings salvation to everyone who believes" (Rom. 1:16).

Some years ago while at a Christian conference, I attended a small-group session on developing and sharing personal testimonials. During the first portion of the workshop, the basic elements of a testimonial were reviewed, including applying a story-line structure, incorporating a scriptural reference, and using compelling vocabulary. After this introduction, we were tasked with writing out our own personal testimonial in under ten minutes, and to do so using no more than 500 words. So, to comply with the exercise, I filled a loose-leaf page with a brief description my life situation before coming to Christ, the *how* and *why* I came to Christ, as well as some of the transformative aspects that occurred afterwards. As requested, I thumbed through my Bible looking for an appropriate Scripture verse and chose, "For he has rescued us from the dominion of darkness and brought us into the kingdom of the Son he loves, in whom we have redemption, the forgiveness of sins" (Col. 1:13-14). As our ten minutes came to an end, we were all paired off and positioned in various places in the room. At that point, I thought that we'd be reading our freshly written stories to each other, but the facilitator threw us a curve ball. Rather than reading, he asked us to put away our coming-to-faith stories, and to share our testimonials from memory. And then he added the challenge of doing so within a one-minute timed interval.

While we were all a bit taken aback by the exercise, the task was easier than I had imagined. Even though my spiel was unrehearsed and time-limited, I found that I was able to use the basic structure which I had planned out, and was pleased to discover that the vocabulary needed to tell parts of my story, including the Scripture quotation, were readily available to my memory. The time constraint forced me to make my points directly and skip the banter. Afterwards, we were provided a chance to rewrite our condensed "Test-a-minutes," as the facilitator called them, into a more polished form, and were given a second one-minute opportunity to share them, this time with a new partner. The whole exercise proved very useful, and one I highly recommend. Not only did the session give me the opportunity to intentionally review the important landmarks of my faith walk, it pushed me to consolidate my thoughts into a concise and easily sharable form. As well, the repeated practice of sharing the testimonial diminished the anxiety around witnessing to faith, and reinforced the transformative role that Jesus has had in my life.

While I don't often directly share my personal testimony in clinical settings, I do try to be generous with my story. To illustrate a point or make a deeper connection with a patient, I try to draw from certain aspects of my life story, including my faith walk. The testimonial exercise that I did has made this easier to do on the fly. Each clinical scenario is different, of course, and requires an ear to the Holy Spirit for discernment, for both content and timing. However, the only patient interactions that I've regretted are the times when I got that still-small-voice nudge to share something, but kept silent instead. So, as important as it is to have a clear worldview understanding of the gospel message, and be able to present an apologetic of our faith, it's also essential that we are able to communicate the more experiential, heart-and-soul elements of our personal faith journey. Sometimes referred to as moving knowledge from the *head* to the *heart*, sharing with patients openly can be invaluable in building trust. This is especially the case when we are caring for dying patients, and assisting them in coming to terms with their death. The end-of-life care of patients is enhanced when we are open to the heart issues at play, particularly as we bring our faith to bear on the complex matters of medical stewardship and palliative care engagement.

MEDICAL STEWARDSHIP IN END-OF-LIFE CARE

When we hear the word *stewardship* in day-to-day conversation, it's typically in the context of environmental activism. Or, if we happen to be sitting in a church pew, it often signifies budget time, or a plea to fund some building project or outreach mission. In medicine, the term *stewardship* is most often applied to judicious antibiotic use, and the associated concerns around limiting the development of antimicrobial-resistant organisms. However, the biblical view of medical *stewardship* has implications that extend beyond all of the above, and has to do with our shrewd utilization and management of every resource with which we've been entrusted – including our time, money, abilities, and information – for the glory of God and the betterment of His creation. Considered in this broader sense, medical stewardship represents the intersection between hospital economics, medical expertise, healthcare provision, and our faith in the living God. This is important for us to consider, since, like the servants in the Parable of the Talents (Matt. 25:14-30), we too will be called to give an account for how we've managed our share of resources. It's not necessarily that we'll be thrown into utter darkness to weep and gnash our teeth if we order some unnecessary lab test, or one too many MRI scans, but there are significant responsibilities here for us to take seriously.

According to reports from the Canadian Institute for Health, the costs of healthcare are escalating exponentially, and account for an increasing proportion of our gross domestic product.[6] Medical provision at the end of life is particularly expensive. It's been estimated that the majority of healthcare expenditures per person occur within the last two months of life.[7] This places increasing scrutiny on healthcare provision for the elderly, as well as on other vulnerable members of our society, and has fostered a growing acceptance that assisted suicide may represent an efficient means of countering our skyrocketing healthcare costs. Former Colorado Governor, Richard Lamm, championed such a view, and argued against maintenance of people with serious chronic conditions on the grounds that the care required would beggar the state. In a brash statement for the *New York Times* he said, "Elderly and terminally ill patients have a duty to die and get out of the way...so that our kids can build a reasonable life."[8]

His shocking sentiment is reminiscent of the propaganda of discrimination leveled towards the disabled in pre-Nazi Germany. Circulating advertisements in the financially bankrupt post-WWI Germany warned of the prohibitive costs of caring for those with hereditary defects using the refrain, "Fellow Germans, this is your money, too!" Such deceptive rationalizations eventually allowed for the development of the infamous T4 program, where dozens of Nazi bureaucrats and like-minded doctors organized the mass murder of over 300,000 sanatorium and psychiatric hospital patients deemed unworthy to live. As Uwe Neumaerker, director of the T4 memorial foundation commented, the extermination program is "considered a forerunner of the extermination of European Jews." During the Nuremberg Trials of 1946, the primary defense of the Nazi physicians was that they had done nothing outside of the law of their land. And while this may have been true, the atrocities committed were considered unacceptable, nonetheless. What will be our defense in Canada when our present actions in regards to MAID, or inactions, as the case may be, are "uncovered and laid bare before the eyes of him to whom we must give account"? (Heb. 4:13).

Adam and Eve were placed in Eden to care for and cultivate the garden (Gen. 2:15). In a similar way, we have been placed within the auspices of healthcare, representing our 'garden' of sorts, to care for and thoughtfully cultivate. Considered this way, it behooves us to limit unnecessary costs and do our best with the resources at hand. This is critical, since medical stewardship and economic considerations can not only prevent the wasting of healthcare resources, limit patient exposure to unnecessary therapies, and minimize futile interventions, it can also help protect the vulnerable from being targeted as a burden, and acquiescing to assisted suicide. A collection of cases follow to help illustrate some of these issues and better highlight the challenges of medical stewardship.

A CASE OF FORCED FUTILITY

I was involved in the management of a coronary care unit patient that exemplified, in extreme, some of the challenges related to medical stewardship when faced with the request for futile care. The patient was an East Asian gentleman in his early 70s, who was brought in through the emergency department as a resuscitated cardiac arrest. He was critically ill and on life support when we accepted him to our unit. He appeared older than his stated age, which was likely related to his significant list of comorbidities, including emphysema from long-time smoking and poorly controlled insulin-dependent diabetes mellitus. We were told that he had been found in the bathroom by a family member. Since he remained obtunded without the need for sedation, we suspected that he had been without adequate pulse and pressure for a significant amount of time – too long, we feared, for realistic recovery. Due to the language barrier, communication with the family was difficult from the get-go. It wasn't until the next day that I was able to secure a translator and explain the patient's dire state. I outlined that his prognosis for recovery was very poor and suggested that we would need to consider the timing of life-support withdrawal. None of this seemed to register with the family. They were determined to wait for family members to arrive from out of country before any such decisions were to take place, and repeatedly emphasized they wanted "everything to be done." Days passed as we awaited the family members' arrival, during which time the patient's condition only deteriorated further. Some of the nurses began complaining about the odor of the patient's weeping foot ulcers, which were worsening despite broad-spectrum intravenous antibiotics, and necessitated repeated dressing changes. As part of our due diligence, we consulted neurology to review the case. Their electroencephalogram evaluation and imaging assessments only confirmed a dismal prognosis. When the out-of-town family finally arrived, communications worsened. Instead of agreeing to withdraw therapy as we had suggested, they demanded that we keep going and even intensify our efforts.

"Why not surgery for his oozing feet? Why not an assist device for his failing heart?" they would ask, not accepting our pronouncements that he was brain dead with no chance of recovery.

Despite numerous discussions to explain the patient's poor prognosis, we remained at loggerheads with the family. Finally, to bring a needed end to the patient's protracted dying process, we involved our hospital ethics committee, as well as legal assistance. After repeated meetings and legal pressure, we were able to disconnect the patient's life-support and allow him to die peacefully.

This type of end-of-life drama doesn't happen very frequently, and good thing, too; the patient's intensive care length of stay was unnecessarily protracted and expensive. Nonetheless, it's common to be faced with patients and families who request costly interventions as their disease process worsens – interventions that offer no meaningful benefit, and merely prolong the dying process. We must resist this, and recognize that behind their requests lurk other issues, such as fear of dying on the patient's part, or guilt on the family's part. Our role is to come alongside those involved during these challenging times with comfort and support, and gently address their fears and concerns.

It's important here that we also distinguish between the value of the therapies and the value of the patient. There is a growing utilitarian shift in medicine, which emphasizes *quality of life* over *sanctity of life,* and places vulnerable patients at risk for receiving inadequate care, or worse, being encouraged to consider assisted suicide.[9] This is shameful because patients have inherent worth regardless of their physical or mental condition, age, or functional status. Even patients who have achieved extreme old age or are demented or handicapped in some way are no less image-bearers of God and remain precious in His eyes. As Christian

195

healthcare professionals, we must always uphold the sanctity of life. Our role is to offer proven effective therapies, balancing risks and benefits, while at the same time resist futile interventions without compromising compassionate care.

A CASE OF RISK AND BENEFIT ASKEW

Another patient that I had been involved with illustrates some of the challenges of balancing this risk and benefit. The patient was a former schoolteacher in her late 80s who had, back in her heyday, taught in a one-room schoolhouse. She had been admitted to our neighboring rehabilitation hospital because of increasing difficulties with weakness, declining cognition, and general failure to thrive. Because a heart murmur was noticed during her hospital admission, the admitting physician arranged an echocardiogram, revealing significant aortic valve stenosis. As a result, I was asked to review the case and render a cardiology opinion regarding the need for valve intervention and recommended management options.

Her heart valve was severely stenosed on clinical grounds, to be sure, but what was even more concerning was her marked frailty. Age had reduced her to a little more than a bird, just skin and bones. It was hard to believe that she had been living independently up to this point. So even though I agreed that she had significant valve disease, I didn't think the narrowed valve was the cause of her advanced infirmity and deteriorating condition, nor limiting her in any functional way. To best explain the situation to the patient, I showed her a real-time image of her heart with my hand-held ultrasound, which I performed at her bedside. Later, I drew her a labelled diagram detailing the pertinent issues. Smiling, she placed an A+ in the upper corner of my picture, and told me that my picture would be useful for explaining things to her visiting family.

When I discussed the various interventional options for such a valve, she indicated that she had no interest in having any procedure done. Even though I wasn't actually intending on offering her a valve intervention, her wishes made my recommendation for a non-interventional palliative approach all the easier.

The attending physician seemed satisfied with my assessment, until some days later when he called and asked me to discuss the case with the patient's son, a physician practicing stateside. When I got a hold of the son, he was quite upset with my conservative recommendations, and was adamant that his mother undergo percutaneous transcatheter aortic valve intervention (TAVI) to remedy her stenotic valve. Despite my attempts to reason with him by outlining her frailty, and the long waitlist for the highly demanded procedure, as well as her own stated wishes, he remained resolute in his request. He told me in no uncertain terms that if I wouldn't agree to valvular intervention, he'd find another cardiologist who would, and then hung up the phone.

That was the last I heard about the case until some weeks later, when one of the members of the TAVI team informed me that my patient had been seen by another cardiologist and had agreed to undergo the valve intervention procedure. He described how things had initially gone smoothly until the bioprosthetic valve was deployed. At that point her aorta ruptured and she died suddenly on the table. This sad news confirmed in my mind that just because we can do some intervention, doesn't mean we always should.

Deciding when and when not to intervene with medicines or surgical procedures is a challenging business. It's an art to choose the right patient for the right intervention. We need to weigh and balance the risks and benefits, as well as the need, feasibility, cost, and even availability. There are unavoidable risks inherent with our interventions. Sometimes complications arise, and sometimes these complications can be fatal.

This underscores the importance of being selective about which patient goes for what procedure. This is particularly the case when resources are scarce, such as with organ transplantation. Although there are usually regulating organizations that carefully monitor such interventions to ensure they operate with a fairness policy, healthcare professionals play an important role as well. We need to thoughtfully consider what is in our patient's best interests and what their wishes are, and balance this patient advocacy with medical stewardship.[10] Prayerful consideration is needed, as well as recollection that "the Lord gives wisdom; from his mouth come knowledge and understanding… Then you will understand righteousness and justice and equity, every good path" (Prov. 2:6-9).

A CASE OF CONTENTMENT

A case from our heart function clinic comes to mind that illustrates the importance of patient engagement coupled with procedural decision-making. The patient was a former labourer in his mid-80s, who had been widowed for two years and followed in our specialty clinic for ischemic cardiomyopathy. He had undergone two separate bypass surgeries in the past, as well as numerous percutaneous coronary interventions. But despite his severely reduced left ventricular function, he was doing reasonably well and continuing to live independently without symptoms. When I asked the nurse to see his most recent electrocardiogram, she told me that it was in the Device Clinic, because he was being considered for an ICD implantation. Although I agreed that based on his reduced heart function, he met the criteria for an implantable cardioverter defibrillator (ICD), I wondered if this would be his desire.

During our consultation, I asked him some general questions about how things were going and what occupied his time. He mentioned that he spent his days doing a little reading and watching some television, and occasionally met friends for coffee. When I asked about physical activity and exercise, he proudly informed me that he walked six blocks every day, back and forth to the cemetery, where his wife was buried. He told me that he had purchased a double plot, had already had his gravestone engraved, and was now "just waiting for the end date." I then explained that because of his poor heart function, he would be a candidate for a specialized pacemaker that could deliver a shock to the heart if needed. I demonstrated on his chest where the pulse generator pocket would be placed, and how the wires would sit in the heart chambers to defibrillate the heart. Although his initial response was agreeable, when I explained that the rationale for having such a device was to prevent sudden cardiac death, his countenance changed.

Shaking his head, he said, "But I'm not afraid of dying, Doc. I know where I'm going. And besides, it's awfully lonely here on my own without my Elizabeth. We almost made our diamond anniversary… we were married 59 years before she died."

I asked him if he had any family, to which he replied that he didn't, that their one son had been killed in car accident over 40 years ago. Aside from a few surviving friends, he confessed that he spent his time predominantly alone. At that point, I reassured him that the decision to proceed with an ICD was his to make, and his only. Not surprisingly, he declined the device when it was later offered by our electrophysiologist.

Guideline recommendations are useful as far as they go. The trouble is, they don't go far enough. Like the jacklines strung from a ship's bow to stern that allow for safe movement on the deck and reduce man-overboard risk, consensus guidelines can help us navigate complex medical management issues, but they don't remove the importance of thoughtful individualized care. Just because the guidelines specify a certain course of action doesn't mean we necessarily need to follow that course. I've often had to discontinue proven-effective therapy, for example, when the side effects produced interfere with the patient's quality of life. Again, just because we can do something, doesn't mean we should – sometimes end-of-life care can actually be undermined by the availability of life-sustaining interventions. In addition to living in a death-loving and death-obsessed society, ours is also curiously a death-denying and death-defying culture. We need to counter the technological imperative which implies that progress is always a good thing and whatever *can* be done *should* be done. Since longevity in and of itself is not the ultimate good, we aren't obliged to extend life at all costs. As members of God's management team, our concern is sanctity of life, not the idolatry of life. It's important to be mindful that "Whatever you do, work at it with all your heart, as working for the Lord, not for human masters, since you know that you will receive an inheritance from the Lord as a reward. It is the Lord Christ you are serving" (Col. 3:23).

PALLIATIVE CARE AT END-OF-LIFE

My first introduction to palliative medicine was in my teens when my mother was a patient on the cancer ward at the old Jubilee Hospital in Victoria. Although palliative care as a medical specialty was just in its infancy at the time, and the provision of end-of-life care hadn't developed to the extent we have today, the medical staff caring for my mother – and the nurses in particular – managed her symptoms well and responded to her needs in a caring and holistic fashion. On my last day visiting her before she died, she had been having a difficult morning with nausea and emesis. As I entered the room, she kept saying to the nurse, "I just want to die… Why can't I just die?" The nurse, who was patiently holding a kidney basin to my mother's mouth, tried to console and settle her. She placed a facecloth on my mother's forehead, and then seeing me at the doorway, softy said, "There will be time to die, Kathy, that will happen soon enough. But this is the opportunity for you to be with your son. Look, he's come to visit you. Why don't you tell him how much he means to you?" After the nurse motioned for me to come closer, I sat down on the edge of the bed and held my mother's hand. She smiled weakly as she looked up at me. Her dark brown eyes seemed so large and out of place staring up at me from her shrunken body.

After a pause, she said with considerable effort, "Oh, my dear... sorry for being such a mess. It's a hard time, but you'll see... life will still be good, even after I'm gone... I love you, son, and am so proud of you... so very proud."

Those were important words for me to hear, words that I often re-play. Although seeing her in such a state was difficult for me, and the last good-bye is the hardest one to say, I wouldn't have traded that moment for the world. It was a sacred time.

Suffering is a complex, multifaceted experience, often involving an array of physical, emotional, and existential symptoms. The goals of palliative care medicine are not only to relieve physical discomfort with expert pain and symptom control, but also to broadly respond to the emotional and spiritual needs of the patient and their family. This kind of holistic proven-effective therapy has been shown to enhance patient's quality of life, mood, and even survival.[11] Relative to my specialty of cardiology, which adds handsomely to healthcare costs in Canada, palliative care medicine is not expensive. In fact, palliative care has actually been shown to decrease overall healthcare costs by enabling patients to spend more time at home with reduced hospital lengths of stay.[12] It's affordable medicine that places value on the dying process, and is an ideal mission field for Christian care and witness.

A CASE OF PURPLE APPENDAGES

One of my patients who benefited from palliative care was a retired nurse originally from Ireland, who I had followed for many years. She was in her mid-70s and suffered from end-stage valvular heart disease. Diagnosed with rheumatic fever as a child, she had undergone three separate open-heart surgeries in her lifetime. Despite this, she had developed severe pulmonary hypertension with secondary right-sided heart failure and cyanotic lips and fingertips. Although she had been placed on home oxygen and maximal medical therapy, she required frequent hospital readmissions to treat her fluid-overloaded state. Her obvious physical findings made her an ideal candidate for bedside teaching. She seemed to enjoy the attention of such interactions, and was always pleased to show the students her "purple appendages," as she called them, for their learning benefit. She was well-aware that she was no longer a surgical candidate, and had entered into the latter stages of her illness.

During her last hospital admission, it wasn't just her lips and hands that were blue; so, too, was her mood and outlook. We hadn't consulted palliative care services on prior admissions because of concerns raised that she would become demoralized. However, during this last admission, I broached the topic with her and she agreed that it might be a good idea. And sure enough it was. Her spirits brightened considerably after the team reviewed her case and adjusted her analgesics. Even her attempts to mobilize improved.

"They've made out-patient homecare arrangements for me. So, I have to strengthen my legs, if I'm going to do that two-stair walk-up in front of my place," she told me as she hobbled back from the bathroom with her oxygen tank balanced on her walker.

Then she surprised me even further by calmly saying that she wanted to get busy planning her funeral. Knowing from prior conversations that I played in a worship band, she asked me about song choices.

"Nothing with too much rock or rap," I said with a smile, and then suggested, "how about In Christ Alone. It's got a wonderful Irish melody and beautiful creedal lyrics."

Before she was discharged home, I had a chance to pray with her and give her a Scripture Script, which read, "Therefore we do not lose heart. Though outwardly we are wasting away, yet inwardly we are being renewed day by day" (2 Cor. 4:16). I received a card from her family some months later thanking me for my care and witness, and saying that she had died peacefully at home, surrounded by her family members.

Palliative care is good medicine. Unfortunately, only an estimated 30% of Canadians who are dying receive proper palliative care. As for palliative homecare, which my patient received, things are even worse. Only 15 per cent of patients have early access to palliative homecare, even though the majority would benefit.[13] This under-representation of palliative care in our healthcare system is complicated by the general confusion as to what the care actually entails. Even fellow physicians get mixed up on this. The widespread use of assisted suicide euphemisms, such as *death with dignity*, *compassionate dying*, and *medical assistance in dying*, have added to this confusion. Some terms are particularly unclear. For example, the medical intervention referred to as *palliative sedation* sounds much like *terminal sedation*, even though the two represent polar opposites of care. Palliative sedation is a technique of inducing a coma in a dying patient with intractable pain. It's a rarely required intervention, and most often done as a temporizing measure. However, *terminal sedation*, by contrast, is a form of euthanasia, carried out with the express purpose of precipitating death in a patient. It's a one-way ticket to death and can be performed in Canada even if the person requesting it isn't even dying. Matters become further befuddled by use of the term, *terminal palliative sedation*, which was propagated by the Quebec Assembly during their political maneuvering. These rhetorical devices have been popularized by those advocating for euthanasia because they are more palatable to our cultural sensibilities, and can better foster agreement. As Margaret Somerville wisely observed, this has led to "legalizing euthanasia through confusion."

As a result, many have come to equate palliative care with assisted suicide, even though the two are diametrically opposed. While palliative care places value on the comfort and care of those dying, euthanasia devalues the dying process and robs patients and their families of potentially life-enriching opportunities of connection and support. As Gilbert Meilaender says, "euthanasia misses the irony that we are attempting to master the very event that announces our lack of mastery."[14] With the shortage of palliative care, many dying patients unfortunately see assisted suicide as their only option. Consequently, euthanasia is effectively undermining palliative care in Canada, and is resulting in its decline rather than promoting its development. Certainly the hospice-style palliative care which we have in Canada is virtually unknown in the Netherlands, where euthanasia has been long-practiced. Our goal is to alleviate suffering, not annihilate the sufferer. Palliative care medicine needs to be further developed and expanded to better address suffering during the dying process; it should not be replaced by lethal injection.

A CASE OF FISH AND FAMILY

The following case of a dying patient illustrates how we might intercept the provision of assisted suicide by providing intentional relational support for patients during moments of vulnerability. The patient was a former heavy-duty mechanic in his mid-70s with long-standing emphysema, who was transferred to the cardiology ward following a complicated heart attack. After my colleague briefed me on the case, relaying that the patient had presented late with an extensive anterior myocardial infarction, ventricular tachycardia, congestive heart failure, acute kidney injury, and aspiration pneumonia, superimposed on his chronic lung disease... I responded, "But he's otherwise doing well, right?" Not so. His aspiration pneumonia had produced a severe pneumonitis causing significant deterioration in his already limited respiratory function. So severe that the patient wasn't expected to survive the hospitalization.

When he arrived on the ward, he was receiving a diuretic infusion, as well as low-dose inotropic support, and was on a non-rebreather mask to help maintain his oxygen saturations. After I introduced myself, he blurted out, "I'm sick and tired of all these tubes and wires. Let's face it, Doc, there's no point in going on. I just wanna die... Gimme the injection and get it over with!"

The *injection* that he was referring to, of course, was the lethal thiopental/pancuronium cocktail used for physician-assisted suicide in our hospital. Although I had no intention of complying with his request, I diverted attention away from that particular battle by sitting next to him and saying with a smile, "Well, before we just *get it over with*, let me chat with you a bit, and ask you a few questions."

After going over some of his medical issues, I asked him about his background and family. He told me that he had been divorced many years prior and had no children. His only close family were his two sisters, living on Vancouver Island. Using that as a point of connection, I asked him where they lived in particular, and informed him that I was originally from the Island and knew it well. His face lit up when I mentioned that I had graduated from high school in Port Alberni, and he told me that the Alberni inlet was one of his favorite fishing destinations. I confessed that I wasn't much of a fisherman, and made him smile when I relayed how I once caught a trout using bacon as bait and a fishing line tied to my leg. At that point, he proudly told me about the time he got third place at the annual Salmon Festival with a thirty-pound Chinook. After I joked about needing to see a photo to believe that story, I discussed with him our treatment plan, and emphasized the importance of informing his sisters about his hospitalization, and that they should visit.

Although we didn't make any noticeable improvement in his kidney function over the next few days, his mood brightened considerably. Even when his condition worsened, he didn't mention assisted suicide again. His sisters arrived, and brought with them various nephews and nieces, along with a framed photograph of the patient holding his prized Port Alberni salmon.

"Wow that is a real monster!" I exclaimed, and then teased, "You're sure that's not Photoshop?"

With the family gathered, I took the opportunity to review the gravity of his condition and the limitations of our treatment options. Then I raised the possibility of transferring him to our palliative care ward. The patient was initially reluctant with this suggestion, but when I outlined the specialized comfort care he could receive there, and reassured him that I would still visit him daily, he agreed with the transfer.

During my visits over the next number of days, his condition steadily worsened. He appeared quite comfortable, but in time become less and less able to speak, and later still, less responsive. When I was informed that he had finally died, I made my way over to the palliative ward to pronounce him. His room was filled to capacity with family and friends. The two sisters were sitting at the foot of the bed and embraced me as I entered the room, introducing me to the assembly. I maneuvered my way over to the head of the patient's bed and slowly removed the oxygen mask from his face. I stood there quietly and briefly held his hand, before taking a seat on the windowsill. After a period of silence, some of the family members started to speak in whispers, then in quiet conversation. Within minutes the stories started; first tender and tearful, but later amusing, and some even comical. There was a general mix of tears and laughter as the family shared memories of their deceased loved one. It was a prime example of *good grief,* which wouldn't have occurred had we carried out his initial request for assisted suicide.

CONCLUDING REMARKS

A *good death,* in a God-honoring sense, is the completion of a life journey, where that life is valued to the end and God decides on the end point. Palliative care plays a central role in facilitating this and, ideally, should be incorporated early in a patient's management trajectory. Rather than having a sharp demarcation between so-called *active treatment* ending and palliative care beginning, it would be helpful for patients and their families to have access to palliative care expertise early on in the time course of serious illness. In this way, as the debility of the disease progresses, the palliative component can be increased to allow a smooth transition from curative to comfort efforts. We can be part of this process by coming alongside our patients and their families, and providing them with support and encouragement as they come to terms with their disease, and ultimately, their death. Rather than accepting the impoverished solution of assisted suicide, we need to remind patients of their value at every level of their disease progression, up to and including their dying days. In this way, loved ones are given the opportunity to make plans for the future, and take part in a healthier grieving process.[15]

Disease and suffering are not ends in themselves. If biblical revelation is suppressed from consideration, it's certainly understandable how feelings of abandonment and despair can enter into the experience of disease and dying. Any eschatology shaped in the exclusion of God is a bankrupt one, and can't bear the burden of facing the abyss. While those who hold fast to a secular eschatology may view their lifeline on a superficial horizontal plane, beginning at birth and ending in death, punctuated by raw deals of suffering along the way, this is delusional thinking. Reality is not this way. So, to keep our faith in our medical practice, we need to consider God's eternal timeline. It's important for us to appreciate that our lives operate on a slope that begins prior to birth and extends ever upwards beyond the grave. Only such an understanding can provide a proper perspective to disease and the dying process. With eternity in mind, times of suffering become relatively small, and are no longer raw deals to complain about, but rich opportunities to witness God's power. As C. S. Lewis suggested, "They say of some temporal suffering, 'No future bliss can make up for it' not knowing that Heaven, once attained, will work backwards and turn even that agony into a glory."[16] As we view our vocational calling in the light of this eternal reality, we can more fully appreciate not only the gift of every working week, but also the preciousness of every person on our patient rosters, and the opportunity of every relational interaction in our day.

SUMMARY POINTS – RESTORATION

1. God has promised an eternal destiny of complete and triumphant restoration of all things

2. Our cultural eschatology is materialistic and fearful

3. Fasting as a spiritual discipline can help guard against secular materialism

4. Rather than having a pick-and-choose approach to Scripture, the Bible needs to be understood as a unified, unfolding and progressive grand narrative

5. Being generous with our story and developing our testimonials can help make valuable connections with patients and foster Christian witness

6. Medical stewardship in end-of-life care can help keep our efforts focussed on patient needs and guard us from considering that longevity is the primary end goal for patient management

7. Palliative care medicine places value on the dying process and is an ideal mission field for Christian care and witness

Questions for Reflection and Discussion

1. Are there portions of Scripture or certain biblical doctrines that you have struggled with? How have you resolved these?

2. Have you ever tried fasting? If so, was it helpful as a spiritual discipline? If not, why not?

3. Do you accept the ultimate destiny of humanity as laid out in the biblical eschatology of Heaven, Hell, and judgement? How might you convince a non-believer of their reality?

4. Have you had experiences that force you to consider your own mortality? How have you dealt with them? Are you prepared to die?

5. What is your ultimate metaphysical commitment for explaining reality? Can you defend this?

6. How do you know things and how do you *know* that you know them?

7. What is your moral standard for addressing issues in medical ethics?

8. Have you shared aspects of your story with patients? How was this received?

9. Have you shared your personal testimony before? Have you had the opportunity but neglected to do so? Why was this the case?

10. Have you been involved with patient therapy or interventions that seemed futile? What could have been done differently?

11. How do views of the *quality of life* versus the *sanctity of life* differ

and conflict?

12. Have you been involved in palliative care cases? What benefits of palliative care medicine have you witnessed?

13. How do you think the provision of MAID has affected palliative care practice in Canada?

CHAPTER NOTES

1. Lewis, C. S. *Mere Christianity*. San Francisco: Harper San Francisco, 2001, 38–39.

2. Bahnsen, G.L. *Always Ready: Directions for Defending the Faith*. Covenant Media Press, 1996.

3. Law, William. *A Serious Call to a Devout and Holy Life*. Whitaker House, 1996.

4. Piper, John. *A Hunger for God: Desiring God through Fasting and Prayer*. Crossway, 2013.

5. Fung, Jason. *The Complete Book of Fasting: heal your body through intermittent, alternate day, and extended fasting*. Victory Belt Publishing, 2016.

6. *Canadian Institute for Health Information Annual Report*, 2019.

7. Fassbender, K., Fainsinger RL, Carson M, Finegan BA. *Journal of Pain and Symptom Management*. 2009 Jul;38(1):75-80.

8. https://www.nytimes.com/1984/03/29

9. Capone, R.A. Grimstad, J. "Futile-care Theory in Practice: a look at the law in Texas." *National Catholic Bioethics Quarterly* 14.4 (Winter 2014); 619-24.

10. Bischoff, K., O'Riordan, D.L., Marks, A.K., et al. "Care Planning for In-patients Referred for Palliative Care Consultation." *JAMA Internal Medicine* 2018; 178:48.

11. *New England Journal of Medicine*. 2010 Aug 19; 363 (8):733-42.

12. Hughes, S.L., Cummings J, Weaver F, et al. "A randomized trial of the cost effectiveness of VA hospital-based home care for the terminally ill." *Health Services Research*. 1992; 26:801–17.

13. Morrison, S. "A National Palliative Care Strategy for Canada." *Journal of Palliative Medicine*. 2017 Dec 1; 20(Suppl. 1): S-63–S-75.

14. Meilaender, Gilbert. "Living life's End." *First Things*, May 2005.

15. Gibbs, J.S. *Heart* 2002;88: Suppl 2 (36).

16. Lewis, C.S. *The Great Divorce*. London: MacMillan, 1946, 64.

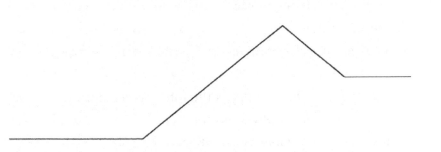

PRACTICING IN THE PRESENCE OF GOD

"Therefore, be imitators of God, as dearly loved children; and walk in
the way of love, just as Christ also loved us and gave himself for us"
Ephesians 5:1-2

The contemporary practice of medicine is a challenging business. The
vastness of the medical need-to-know database is growing exponentially
in every field, and has driven medical education into a hyperspecialized
mode. Even just trying to remain current in a single area of a subspe-

cialty can be a mind-numbing task. Coupled to this volume-overload challenge is the growing complexity of bioethical issues with their interwoven political agendas and inescapable legal matters. Driven by the fear of litigation, diagnostic acumen is being replaced by defensive medical practice. The literature is rife with case reports detailing successful lawsuits against physicians who "didn't order the test."[1] Aware of this danger, contemporary practitioners often shy away from making medical decisions on the basis of careful clinical assessment, and instead order expensive and often unnecessary investigations.[2] In the process, time spent with patients is often reduced, and opportunities for therapeutic connections lost. When clinical interactions do occur, the rapport-building prospects are often hampered by the juxtaposition of laptop between practitioner and patient. Although top-down lip service is often paid to the importance of patient-centered care, in the hectic day-to-day maelstrom of medicine, the patient can get easily sidelined and sometimes even forgotten. These issues are likely to escalate as advanced technology assumes a greater position in healthcare.

Artificial intelligence (AI) has arrived at the threshold of medical practice and is positioned to revolutionize the diagnosis, treatment and delivery of medicine,[3] However, the promised benefits of AI are often overshadowed by alarmist warnings as to the detrimental effects of its development. From Stanley Kubrick's 2001: A Space Odyssey to Todd McAulty's Robots of Gotham, popular culture is rife with the potential negative aspects of AI, imagining future dystopias and the rise of killer robots. In a 2016 interview with BBC, Stephen Hawking warned that "the development of full artificial intelligence could spell the end of the human race." Even tech giants, such as Microsoft's Bill Gates, Tesla designer Elon Musk, and Apple co-founder Steve Wozniak, share similar predictions of how AI may deleteriously affect society. Frenzied by the Covid-19 pandemic, and tired by repeatedly sounding the climate

216

doomsday siren, the media machine has set its sights on AI, reporting predictions of how advanced technology will cause calamitous job losses and deleterious disruptions of communities.[4] So, although the positive applications of big data, cognitive computing, and deep learning have created a degree of excitement in the medical community, many remain fearful as to the potential harm AI will produce in healthcare.

The concerns about AI in healthcare are not unfounded. In addition to significant developmental costs, data privacy issues, and cybersecurity threats, several predict that AI will reduce clinic productivity, increase health system bureaucracy, and turn healthcare professionals into data managers.[5] Increased computer reliance in medicine has been cited as not only an obstacle to patient care, but the related frustrations and time demands are felt to be a contributing factor for the rise of physician burnout and climbing suicide rates.[6] As well, there are indications that computers may overshadow the human side of medicine by replacing medical staff and reducing opportunities for personal interactions and care. Examples of this include: Chatbox therapists programmed to diagnose anxiety and depression, therapy robots teaching social skills to children with autism, "Bots" with humanoid faces providing assistance and companionship in nursing homes, and "Robo-docs" gliding between hospital beds to assess patients under the joystick control of doctors at a distance.[7]

While these are valid concerns, adopting advanced technologies in medicine doesn't need to mean the end of bedside manners or compassionate care. We should proceed with caution, to be sure, but proceed we must. As Stewart Brand said, "Once a new technology rolls over you, if you're not part of the steamroller, you're part of the road."[8] Living out our faith in the sphere of medicine is less about trying to hold back time and tide, and more about looking for opportunities to shine God's light in dark places. After all, it's not a competition between computers and clinicians. Computers may be able to mimic human-like thought processes, such as data analysis and self-correction, but they remain programmed computers, nonetheless, and not human beings created in the image of God. They may be able to outperform humans at certain automated tasks such as data mining, information integration, novel drug discovery, and even diagnostic performance and disease prediction, but nothing will ever replace humans taking care of humans. The activities of computers, no matter how advanced, remain programmed, imitative, and algorithmic, not intuitive, contemplative or creative, and incapable of compassion. A computer cannot understand what it has been provided to learn, nor the meaning of the output, but must rely upon our interpretation and ability to make sense of the data.[9] Therefore, expert knowledge of pathophysiology and clinical presentation that physicians acquire over the course of their training and career will remain vital. It's been said, "The computer is incredibly fast, accurate, and stupid. Man is unbelievably slow, inaccurate, and brilliant. The marriage of the two is a force beyond calculation."[10] In brief, computers and clinicians occupy distinct roles. Although there may be overlap between the two, it's best to consider this interface as augmented intelligence, and focus our attention on exploiting the efficiencies of advanced technology in order to better serve our patients.

Never before has the technical expertise of medicine so desperately needed a priestly counterpart of compassionate care than in our present era. The impersonal systems of healthcare, however efficient, are incapable of meeting the existential needs of patients. Patients are often left without a clear understanding of their diagnosis, and sometimes without even knowing who their doctor is. When faced with the spectre of disability and disease, questions like, "What's wrong with me?" "How will it affect me?" "What can be done?" quickly multiply into fear and anxiety if left unanswered. In the absence of supportive relationships, it's no wonder that many suffer from identity crisis. In such times of distress, it's easy to see how meaning in suffering can be elusive, and how feelings of despair and defeat can dominate the clinical experience. It's like a double injury: the first being the physical suffering, and the second the accompanying existential suffering. Our practitioner-patient relationships remain critically important to address these needs. As Dr. John Noseworthy wisely observed, "the patient–physician relationship is fundamental to the future of health care. So, we need to invest in it once again. Healing begins when patients and their physicians build trust – a process that often takes time, especially when the patient's health and future are in jeopardy. There is no app for that."[11] This is why the need for expert clinical skills, top-notch teaching ability, and compassionate care will not diminish with the further application of advanced technology in healthcare, but become even more important. As followers of Christ, we are ideally equipped to address the deeper concerns. By taking time to develop relationships with our patients, we can meet a growing need for compassionate care in the increasingly technology-dominated sphere of healthcare.

To fully embrace this priestly calling of medicine, it's important that we operate from a godly place of strength, centered squarely on a living faith in Christ. This requires that we nurture our own spiritual health and wellbeing. Like first donning one's own oxygen mask before assisting others, in order to be salt and light to our patients, we need to be sure and certain in what we believe. Before we can honestly address a patient's misplaced identity, for example, we need to be clear as to where our identity lies. Unless our needs for significance, security, and acceptance are founded on the solid ground of Christ, we will have little to offer those who are struggling with identity crisis or confusion. Medical credentials, collegial kudos, and bank statements won't suffice. Only a core identity formed around a personal relationship with Jesus will provide the needed perspective to recognize identity struggles in the clinical setting, and speak creational truth into them. Likewise, our ability to come alongside our patients in their times of distress will be hampered unless we have worked out our own theology of suffering. When facing trials in our professional work and personal life, it's essential we understand that we're not alone, and that God has not abandoned us to our suffering, but meets us there. Bolstered in this way, we'll be better equipped to identify opportunities where we might bring meaning into a patient's existential suffering, gently steer them from false remedy, and witness a future of hope rather than one of only futility and defeat.

For medicine to advance in holistic fullness, it's critical that we reclaim the priestly role of the healthcare practitioner. No longer can we rationalize a nominal Christian engagement in the medical sphere by compartmentalization of our faith into sacred Sundays and secular weekdays. The Sabbath was made for man, to be sure, but our calling is to live out our faith on a daily basis. We can't stand idle as our faith gets attacked by secular agendas or forced into the realm of personal preference. It's important to appreciate that we are ambassadors of Christ in all that we do, and co-labourers with the Holy Spirit in every activity of our day. As ambassadors, then, our faith needs to be manifested in personal commitment to objective public reality. This means that we take seriously our role in the body of Christ. As per Aesop's "union gives strength" fable, it's harder to break a bundle of sticks than a single branch. So, too, we'll have firmer resolve to stand up against the devil's schemes in healthcare if we know we're not alone. Rather than allowing our faith to be privatized or dismissed, we need to be bold in our faith, and actively involved with our local church, as well as with para-church organizations working for the Kingdom.

To keep faith in medicine, we need to keep faith in mind. The ambition of this book was to provide a practical approach to how we might live out our Christian faith commitment on a day-to-day basis, in the challenging sphere of secular healthcare. The spiritual disciplines profiled are offered as examples of how we might guard ourselves from secular thought, and allow for astute recognition of the counter-narratives that are operative in the medical culture within which we're immersed. The use of clinical cases is an attempt to demonstrate the practical utility of Christian witness in the clinical setting, and illustrate an approach to patient interaction with suggested word choice, style, and content. In all of this, my hope is that this work might provide encouragement for all Christian healthcare professionals, so we "do not grow weary in doing good" (Gal. 6:14).

Our work in healthcare is Kingdom work. Let us not forget that despite the chaos of our present moment, God is present and working all things for good. Solomon said that "God has set eternity on the hearts of men" (Eccl. 3:11). As we walk down the hospital hallways and negotiate through gurneys in the emergency room, let us do so with an eye on eternity. Let us live out our professional lives worthy of the guaranteed inheritance that we have in Christ. So, when it's all said and done, and we come face to face with our Redeemer, may we hear the words, "well done, good and faithful servant" (Matt. 25:21).

"Finish, then, Thy new creation; Pure and spotless let us be; Let us see Thy great salvation perfectly restored in Thee; Changed from glory into glory; Till in Heav'n we take our place; Till we cast our crowns before Thee; Lost in wonder, love, and praise."[12]

Chapter Notes

1. Studdert, D.M., Mello MM, Sage WM, Des Roches CM, Peugh J, Zapert K, et al. "Defensive medicine among high-risk specialist physicians in a volatile malpractice environment." *Journal of the American Medical Association.* 2005; 293:2609–17.
2. "The Demise of the Physical Exam." *New England Journal of Medicine* 2006; 354:548.
3. Krittanawong, C. "Artificial Intelligence in Precision Cardiovascular Medicine." *Journal of the American College of Cardiology.* 2017 May 30; 69(21):2657-2664.
4. Interview with Kai Fu Lee. *Fortune* January 10, 2019.
5. Wright, A. A. and Katz, I.T. *New England Journal of Medicine.* 2018; 378:309-311.
6. "Medscape National Physician Burnout & Suicide Report 2020: The Generational Divide."
7. "A role for robots in caring for the elderly." *The Network.* May 16, 2016 (https://newsroom.cisco.com/feature)
8. Brand, S. (1987) in *Shaping the Network Society: the New Role of Civil Society in Cyberspace.* MIT Press, 2004, 43.
9. "Deconstructing the diagnostic reasoning of human versus artificial intelligence." *Canadian Medical Association Journal.* January 06, 2020 192 (1) E17.
10. Cherne, Leo (1977) in Garland, R. *Microcomputers and Children in the Primary School. Falmer Publishers,* 1982.
11. Noseworthy, J. "The Future of Care – Preserving the Patient–Physician Relationship." *New England Journal of Medicine.* 2019; 381:2265-2269.
12. Charles Wesley. *Love Divine, All Love Excelling.*